Richardson, John

The Philosophical Principles of the Science of Brewing

ISBN: 978-1-948837-16-3

This classic reprint compilation was produced from digital files in the Google Books digital collection, which may be found at http://www.books.google.com. The artwork used on the cover is from Wikimedia Commons and remains in the public domain. Omissions and/or errors in this book are due to either the physical condition of the original book or due to the scanning process by Google or its agents.

John Richardson's **The Philosophical Principles of the Science of Brewing** was originally published in 1788 (York).

Townsends
PO Box 415, Pierceton, IN 46562
www.Townsends.us

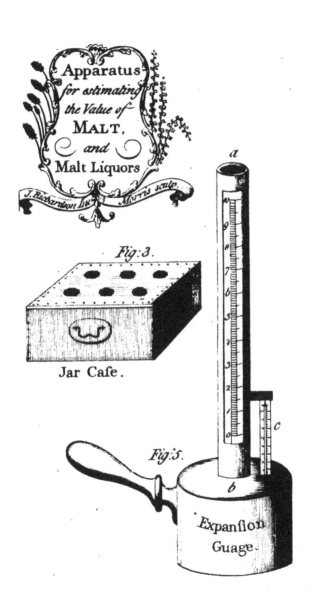

Apparatus for estimating the Value of MALT, and Malt Liquors

J. Richardson inv.ᵗ   Morris sculp.

Fig:3.

Jar Case.

Fig:5.

Expansion Guage.

THE
PHILOSOPHICAL PRINCIPLES

OF THE

Science of Brewing;

CONTAINING

THEORETIC HINTS on an improved Practice

OF

BREWING MALT-LIQUORS;

AND

Statical Estimates of the *Materials* for 'rewing,

OR

A TREATISE on the APPLICATION

AND

USE of the SACCHAROMETER;

BEING

New Editions, corrected, of those Treatises,

With the Addition of

The USE of the SACCHAROMETER
SIMPLIFIED, &c. &c.

By JOHN RICHARDSON.

YORK:

PRINTED BY A. WARD, FOR G. G. AND J. ROBINSON,
PATER-NOSTER-ROW, LONDON; T. BROWNE, HULL;
C. ELLIOT, EDINBURGH; LUKE WHITE, DUBLIN; AND
T. WHITE, CORK.

MDCCLXXXVIII.

PREFACE.

THAT the *brewing bufinefs* is of the utmoft importance to Great Britain, is fufficiently evinced, by the very confiderable portion of the public revenue thence arifing; by its commercial advantages, as an article of trade; and by its effential utility to individuals, whether we confider it as producing the common beverage of every table, from the higheft nobility to the loweft mechanic, or view it in the more beneficial light of aiding, promoting, or fupplying that hale vigor and corporeal ftrength obfervable in the lower part of the inhabitants of this kingdom, by which they are enabled to fuftain a life of amazing labor and fatigue, with alacrity and perfeverance. That a bufinefs of fuch public concern and private utility, fhould not have made an earlier progrefs towards general perfection, may feem a matter of furprize to any one who has only taken a flight view of the

a 2

fubject;

subject; but, when it is considered, that we are apt to estimate objects by the difficulty of acquisition, rather than by the value of possession; that in proportion as they are familiarized to us, they become of less consideration in our ideas; that to make them *common*, is to bring them into *contempt*; it were no longer to be wondered at, that the brewing business has so generally escaped a liberal investigation, when the pretension to a competent knowledge of it, in every person who keeps a common victualling-house, and in almost every servant girl who engages to do the drudgery of a farmer's kitchen, has rendered an art of the first national importance, an object of the veriest insignificance, and not seldom of ridicule and contempt, considered as a scientific subject.

Hence it is that the *brewing of malt-liquors*, an art more complicated in its processes, and more delicate in the criterions which mark the several stages of its various operations than, perhaps, that of producing any other domestic liquor in

the

the world, is generally entrusted to the care and superintendence of persons wholly ignorant and illiterate, to the great detriment of both the produce and the employer.

In the country, this is almost universally the case, the acting brewer being no other than one of the common servants of the office, preferred to this charge on the sole consideration of his having been employed in a brewhouse somewhat longer than his fellows; whence arise those disagreeable qualities so often complained of in the beer of many common brewhouses; to the discredit of the practitioner, and the disgrace of the profession, whilst *home-brewed beer* is extolled and preferred, in terms equally reproachful and injurious to both.

That many private families pique themselves on the acknowledged excellence of their malt-liquor, made by a servant wholly unacquainted with the *principles of brewing*, is certainly true, and thence is inferred the non-existence of any difficulty in the art, beyond the mechanical

compre-

comprehenfion of fuch an artift; but it muft be remembered, on this occa-fion, that the fame beer which is the private gentleman's boaft, would be the common brewer's ruin. The gentleman confiders the *quality*, not the *coft* of his liquor; fo that, in allowing an abundant quantity of materials, to make it *potent*, and a fufficient length of time, to bring it into *condition*, he, in a great meafure, guards againft the blunders of an ignorant operator; for a very rich extract of the principal ingredients may, after a con-fiderable time, become a tolerable liquor, though it fhould have been very errone-oufly formed; which at once accounts for the difference often obfervable in the products of the private and public brewer, though both may be of equal capacity and knowledge in their profeffion.

Oppofed to this imaginary excellence, the common brewer has difficulties of a much greater magnitude to contend with. He has to provide for a tax of 50 to 80 per cent. on the materials, at the fame time that he endeavours to produce a fale-able

able commodity, that fhall at once accommodate the palate of the confumer,
and yield an emolument equivalent to the
rifque of his capital. Thefe ends are
only obtainable, to that degree of advantage of which the fubject is capable, from
a knowledge of the principles of brewing,
on which alone depends the very great
difparity of fuccefs frequently experienced
by brewers circumftanced alike in every
other refpect; for fuperior knowledge
will ever accomplifh fuperior advantages,
and it were in vain to expect a lafting
fuperftructure where there is wanting a
firm foundation.

To evince, in the firft place, the national importance of this bufinefs, it were
only neceffary to premife, that the duties
on beer in the year ending July 5th, 1784,
were 1,932,272*l.* 7*s.* 11*d.* to which adding the duty on malt, in the fame term,
amounting to 1,751,334*l.* 10*s.* 10*d.* and
the duty on hops 75,739*l.* 15*s.* 3*d.* we
fhall fee that the amount of the revenue
arifing from, or principally dependent on
the

the brewery, is the enormous fum of 3,759,346 *l*. 14 *s*. 0 *d*. or perhaps near FOUR MILLIONS STERLING per annum; as the hop-duty for that year was under the average amount, and it is very rea-fonable to fuppofe that the duty on malt was in the fame predicament, on account of the high price of barley, and the little inducement there was for keeping up the ufual ftocks.

From this view of the matter, it is evi-dent that the duty immediately charged on beer is more than one half of this very great amount; and it may afford matter of curious fpeculation to be informed, that the *London brewery*, alone, produces about one-fourth of the whole of this duty, as will be feen by the following abftract of the year ending July 5th, 1786:

Strong beer duty	——	£ 526,914	6	1¾
Small —— do.	——	6,524	7	11¾
Table beer do.	——	48,202	13	11½
		£ 581,641	8	1
Deduct				
Malt allowance on ftrong beer		£ 97,276	17	0
do. —— fmall ——		1,848	2	10
		£ 99,124	19	10
Net amount of duty on beer		£ 482,516	8	3

This

This large fum was the produce of 1,519,249¼ barrels of ftrong, 110,890 barrels of fmall, and 374,943 barrels of table beer, the particulars of which will be found in the fubjoined lift of the London brewers, which I have been in-duced to infert as no unacceptable infor-mation to my country readers, and no difhonorable evidence of the prodigious trade of that immenfe capital.

The brewery ftanding thus high in the fcale of the public revenue, the very humble rank which it obtains in the circle of the fciences is the more to be regretted, and ought to be a fpur to the ambition of its profeffors to raife it into the important notice it merits, that it may no longer be the rough rock upon which government builds the bulk of her finance, but become the finifhed co-lumn of the edifice, fo that the fupported and the fupporter may be contemplated with equal admiration.

That this cannot be done without the ferious efforts of individuals to fhake off habitual errors, and emerge from the

b   pro-

profeffional obfcurity of their anceftors,
may be inferred from the volume here
prefented to the public; but to fet the
matter of general improvement in a ftill
lefs problematical light, and at the fame
time to intimate that there are qualities
refident in the materials for brewing
which are only obtainable by a fcientific
intimacy with the fubject, it may not be
improper to take a curfory view of the
practice of the brewhoufe, in fuch parts as
may beft tend to that purpofe.

It were, perhaps, of no importance to
intimate to the brewer, the requifite
qualities of the materials themfelves. Thefe
being objects of his choice, rather than
the produce of his fkill, it may fuffice
that he be able to view them with a difcriminating eye, in order to felect fuch
as poffefs the particular qualities neceffary
to particular purpofes, and to vary them
according to the intended characterifticks
of his liquor, or the feveral occafions of
his practice.

The whole procefs of brewing, from
the entire ftate of the materials to the final
recom-

recompofition of their extracts, may be divided into three fections; omitting to particularize the preparaton of the *grift*, though its extreme fimplicity has not been able to guard it againft popular prejudice, which has been found fo prevalent, that, to anfwer a purpofe which no one has yet fatisfactorily explained, a demonftrable lofs, to a very confiderable amount, is the certain confequence to thofe who adopt it, when a moment's reflection and an eafy experiment, would convince them of its inconfiftency.

I. *Taking the Liquor.*

IN this preliminary part of the procefs, the fkill of the brewer is very much to be exerted, as various malts require various degrees of heat for the more advantageous extraction of their valuable parts, and the greater perfection of the product; to determine on which, will materially reft in the judgment of the operator. Here it is to be obferved, too, that the *firft liquor* inevitably ftamps a characteriftical impreffion on the whole

b 2 gyle;

gyle; and as the complexion of the future product muſt receive a powerful
tincture from this leading principle, ſo an
error once committed in its application,
will ever leave traces of its influence, in
ſpight of the efforts of the moſt judicious
operator. Whence it is evident, how
much the *uſe of the thermometer* ought to
be ſtudied by the brewer, in order to inſure
him that certainty of ſucceſs which he
can by no diſſimilar means obtain. Without this inſtrument, it is impoſſible he
can accommodate his practice to the different qualities of his malts, ſo as to
ſecure to himſelf every obtainable advantage. The diſcrimination of the ſenſes
is limited and irregular. Beyond the
temperature of the body our judgment
of heat cannot reach, and within that
degree it is very incompetent. In this
buſineſs, the variation of a very few
degrees, which the inſtrument only can
determine, produces effects not leſs extraordinary in themſelves, than important
to the intereſt of the brewer. It is here
the foundation is laid of that deſirable
quality

quality *tranfparency*, which, by a proper regulation of heat, according to the quality of the malt, may be procured in a few days, or poftponed to as many weeks or months, agreeable to the convenience of the brewer or the tafte of the confumer.

From thefe confiderations may be inferred the vexatious confequences which often refult from wrong practice herein; and it is a demonftrable truth, that many difgraceful properties of beers have here their origin, which being attributed to other caufes, the operator is induced to perfift in errors, which ever lead to difappointment and lofs.

II. *Boiling of Worts.*

TO a perfon unacquainted with the brewing bufinefs, it would appear almoft incredible that an operation fo fimple as this, fhould have occafioned fuch a diverfity of opinion amongft the practical brewers. Some contend for a *fhort*, others for a *long time*, and there are thofe who obferve *no time at all*, being

guided

guided by certain criterions to judge of the proper period when to *ſtrike* their worts. Theſe, agreeable to their ſeveral intentions, may be all right; on the contrary, they may be all wrong. A particular attention to their ſeveral uſes may be advantageous, though a general adoption of either muſt be prejudicial. According to the qualities the intended gyle is to poſſeſs, ſhould this operation be varied. To ſome beers the *criterion* is eſſential, to others *time* is indiſpenſible; nor are the diſtinguiſhing qualities of the moſt celebrated malt-liquors to be obtained and preſerved, without the ſtricteſt attention to this particular; whence it will not appear at all extraordinary, that the copper often receives a good extract, and turns out a bad wort.

III. *Fermentation.*

OF all the parts of the brewing proceſs, this is at once the moſt difficult to conduct, the moſt ſubject to error, and the moſt important to the intereſt of the brewer. The *preſervative quality*, the *diſtinguiſhing flavor*, the *body*, and *ſpiri-*
tuoſity

tuofity are here to receive their actual existence. Here, again, the *thermometer* muſt be the grand clew to direct the artiſt, fecurely and with certainty, to the feveral intereſting windings of this fubtile and perplexing labyrinth, without which he is in the utmoſt danger of being perpetually bewildered, if not abfolutely loſt. *Chance*, it is true, may fometimes direct him right; but he muſt be a very ignorant traveller who would truſt his fafety, in a dangerous and intricate road, to the fortuitous conduct of fo blind a guide, when he can put himfelf under the guidance of a fafe and experienced conductor. The fuccefs of the brewer, in this article of his procefs, will ever be precarious, without a knowledge of the ufe of the thermometer, in its newly-difcovered mode of application, by which the accidents to which fermentation is extremely liable, and which the niceſt perception of the fenfes cannot frequently difcover, are immediately detected. Whence it may, with great juſtice, be termed the *index* of this extraordinary operation,

which

which at all times points out the several
periods of its progress, and without which
the operator muſt ever be as uncertain of
truth, as he who judges of the time of
day by a watch deprived of its hour-
hand.

To particularize the ſeveral important
properties finally reſulting from a judicious
management of fermentation, it may be
neceſſary to advert to thoſe qualities above
cited, as actually exiſting in, or ulti-
mately derived from it.

Firſt, the *preſervative quality* has but a
partial reſidence in fermentation. Hops,
undoubtedly, furniſh the *preſervative* of
beers; but they can only be conſidered as
ſupplying the ſemina of that quality,
which, by their extraction in the boiling
worts, may be ſaid to be ſown, whilſt
the active powers of a perfect fermentation
are, alone, the genial ſhower and vivify-
ing ray which quicken and mature the
expected product. Several known inſtances ſpeak in confirmation of this,
where beers have had a ſufficient quantity
of this vegetable to have preſerved them.

found

found for two years, and have notwith-
standing come *forward* in two months ;
and that it refults from an ill-condu&ed
fermentation only, is further evinced by
the obfervation, that fuch beers are always
ftale and *bitter* at the fame time, arifing from
an imperfe& union and recompofition of
the feveral parts of the extra&s, which is
the peculiar bufinefs of fermentation to
accomplifh, in the utmoft perfe&ion, under fuch regulations and reftri&ions as lie
beyond the vague procefs of the random
pra&itioner, and the ill-founded hypothefis of the mere fpeculatift.

II. The *diftinguifhing flavor* of malt-
liquors is, alfo, materially refident in this
interefting part of the procefs. The liquor here affumes various flavors, according to the force of, and time of continuance under the a&ion. It is here in a&ual
embryo, and, like heated wax, ready to
receive the minuteft foreign impreffion ;
whence we are cautioned againft accidents
which might prove injurious, and are led
to attempt the improvement of natural
flavors. Thus, by a proper regulation

c   and

and conduct of fermentation, the most pleasing genuine flavors are naturally, as well as some others, by certain adventitious means, obtainable, to any desired degree of perfection.

III. By the *body* of beers, is not to be understood the *strength*, but the consistence, the materiality, if it may be so termed, which is distinguished by the palate into *light, heavy, thin, full, soft, smart*, either of which it is eminently in the power of fermentation to supply, as far as is consistent with the real strength and goodness of the wort. These desirable ends are of the greater import, since *the gratification of the palate* is the first object of the brewer's attention, because it is the first inducement to the disposal of his liquor; *strength* being but a secondary consideration in the estimation of malt-liquors, the goodness of which is ever marked by those great essentials of a saleable commodity, *flavor* and *transparency*, as qualities less easily obtained than *potency*; for it may be in the power of a person to make *strong* beer,

when

when it fhall baffle the utmoft exertion
of his art to make it *pleafant*.

IV. *Spirituofity*, both in its origin and
exiftence, as it relates to the foregoing
article, may be termed the *vital principle*
of malt-liquors, whence they acquire the
power of invigorating the body, and ox-
hilarating the mind. The mere extracts
of the materials, either feverally or in
combination, exhibit no figns of this
principle, till the reciprocal action of
their parts, in fermentation, calls it into
life. It is well known that *muft* * produces no fpirit in diftillation, and every
brewer can tell that the ftrongeft *raw
wort* would have no inebriating effect on
the drinker. Nor is this to be accounted
for, by the fuppofition that certain parts
of the *muft* act on the body as a corrector
of the inebriating quality, but by the
abfolute non-exiftence of fpirituofity,
previous to fermentation ; for the recom-
mixture of the whole component parts of
the wort, after their feparation, &c. by
this action, rather increafes than dimi-
nifhes

c 2

* *Unfermented extracts of fermentable fubjects.*

nifhes its intoxicating power; thence intimating, that fermentation does not *fet
at liberty*, but pofitively *creates* the fpirituous parts of the liquor.

This, then, is the grand field where
the artift is to reap the chief harveft of
his labors. If fermentation, as is evident,
be the only part of the procefs which
realizes the potency of malt-liquors, it
muft thence occur to the moft ordinary
capacity, that every error in this complicated bufinefs, is a real lofs of ftrength to
the beer, and a confequential diminution
of the brewer's profits; on the contrary,
every new advantage obtained therefrom,
is an additional emolument, without in-
creafing the price or diminifhing the quality of his liquor. It is not, however,
to be hence underftood, that *length of
time* conftitutes perfection in this action,
notwithftanding the prevailing opinion, on
this fubject, which has a ftrong tendency
thereto. Fermentation carried beyond a
certain period, defeats its own purpofes,
by proceeding to undo all that it has before done. This period is when the

operation

operation is arrived at fuch a height as to
require the immediate *cleanfing* of the liquor into cafks, a crifis to which no formal rules can pofitively direct, it fometimes happening in the fpace of one day,
fometimes not till the expiration of many,
ever varying according to the ftrength,
the heat, the quantity, and even local
fituation of the fermenting liquor; and
this crifis has fo delicate a relation to the
quality of the fubject, that, in fome particular proceffes, to anticipate, or exceed
it, but a very few hours, would prove
deftructive to the gyle. To avoid both
extremes, with certainty and precifion,
requires a very clear infight into this
perplexing bufinefs; a difficulty which
is now rendered entirely familiar, by the
affiftance of the thermometer, which not
only difcovers an imperfect from a perfect
fermentation, but, with certain concomitant appearances, diftinguifhable by the
perception of the fenfes, points out the
proper period of *cleanfing* to infallible
nicety; at which period, alone, is to be
expected that regular *purgation* in the

cafks,

casks, which equally avoids the *violence* tending to acidity, and the *languor* that produces the most disagreeable vapidity, heaviness, ill flavor, and a train of other evils which do not immediately discover themselves.

———————

FROM the foregoing few strictures, it is easy to conceive, what a number of advantages accrue to a proficient in the art, from well-conducted processes; and how many valuable qualities are lost to the unskilful professor, from the want of a knowledge of *the component parts of the materials, the proper modes of extracting their virtues, the purposes of their combination, and the action and result of their combined powers.* Possessed of this knowledge, the operator is enabled to accommodate, with every assurance of success, the various palates of the consumers, with equal advantage and reputation. If a *mild, sparkling liquor* be preferred, he can produce spontaneous pellucidity, and every principle of perfection, in a few weeks.

weeks. If a *soft, full* beer be required, he knows how to effect this, without adding to his grift, as well as he can give *lightness* and *vinosity*, without diminishing the strength of his liquor. To this knowledge, also, he is indebted for an effectual security against those bugbears of the ignorant operator, *cloudiness, violent fretting, flatness,* &c. &c. whilst it produces an unsolicited extension of trade, with superior liquor, and superior emolument.

To remedy the disappointments and losses resulting from bad practice, and to render this important business of more general utility to the public, and more particular advantage to individuals, is the purpose of the Author, who, by a continued application to the subject, during several years practice and experience, has had the happiness to reduce the brewing science to a plain system, confirmed throughout by the most successful events. His *theory* is not a chimera of the brain, nor his *practice* the child of hypothesis. By a studious attention to a long course

of

of repeated experiments, in the production of every variety of malt-liquor, the *former* is difcovered, which again, with reflected light, illumines the *latter*; fo that by mutual reflection both are eftablifhed and confirmed, to a degree of certainty equal to the utmoft wifhes of the operator.

IT is hoped the reader will find at leaft a partial confirmation of this in the fubfequent fheets, now firft publifhed in a collected form; and that he will do the Author the juftice to believe that the particulars of his fyftem which, for obvious reafons, he withholds from the eye of the public, are not lefs founded in philofophical inveftigation, nor lefs worthy the attention of the enquiring artift.

A

A LIST of the LONDON BREWERS,

With the several Sums of the Strong, Small, and Table Beer brewed by them respectively in the Year ending at Midsummer, 1786.

A	Barrels of Strong	Barrels of Small	Barrels of Table Beer
Thomas Allen	17,581	106	
William Allen	105		7,260
Mary Amey	10,802	19	9,055
Amos Asquith	4,220	3,018	1,922
Joseph Asquith	2,541	315	1,166
George Ainsworth	801	171¾	2,092
John Armstrong	203	263¼	627
Haggar Allis		1,346	3,903
B			
Francis Bullock	20,364	839	55
Edward Bond	5,991	966	9,408
Timothy Bentley	1,944		2,953
Thomas Bentley	1,076		7,110
Richmond Barker	3,703		3,976
John Barnet	1,716	3,567	
Joseph Butler	1,072		1,037
John Butcher	1,313		2,010
Peter-Thomas Blackwell	788	3,385	
William Briand	408	201	4,582¼
Robert Bradfield	61		1,442
Robert Brown	26		116
Joseph Bristow	3		838
C			
Felix Calvert	117,737	104	
John Calvert	93,774	4,512	106
Thomas Cokar	32,733	1,463	397
Edward Clarke	8,958	1,378	31
John Curtis	10,468	8,111	3
Benjamin Cape	6,891		17,478
John Charrington	10,644	3,504	11,817
Robert Kilby Cox	1,103	49	12,238
Carried over	357,026	33,318½	101,622½
	d		Brought

	Barrels of Strong	Barrels of Small	Barrels of Table Beer
Brought over	357,026	33,318½	101,622¼
Jeremiah Clegg	988	——	3,646
Robert Chapman	652	564	1,394
William Carpenter	683	——	1,371
William Cox	——	——	559
John Cotton	11	419	402
John McCarty	——	5	36
Thomas Carpenter	65	——	353
William Cade	4	——	315
John Carfe	110	1,514	——
John Cowell	——	——	1,804
James Cove	——	——	406
D			
Edmund Dawfon	44,282	1,161	——
Jofeph Dickenfon	32,103	1,083	438
Rivers Dickenfon	24,837	1,044½	——
Oliver Dickenfon	8,497	——	4,567
John Dyer	2,783	2,271¾	1,376
George Davis	2,183	800	1,092
Oliver Davis	987	1,129	3,933
Thomas Drane	571	——	4,595
Elizabeth Deyman	619	928	14
Thomas Days	1,074	8	2,293
John Dore	101	——	2,017
E			
John Edmonds	411	——	8,514
Jofeph Ellerbeck	352	——	1,621¼
William Edwards	74	——	3,151
John Evans	36	4	112
Robert Enftone	178	——	1,142
Jofeph Eldia	——	386	947
John Ellis	——	7	66
F			
Thomas Faffet	44,108	642	——
Felix Feaft	17,354	42	282
John Fifher	1,519	——	883
John Farmer	289	——	8,603
John Farne	4	——	664
William Flack	40	——	557
John Forfter	——	——	278
Carried over	541,941	45,326¼	159,053½
			Brought

	Barrels of Strong	Barrels of Small	Barrels of Table Beer
G Brought over	541,941	45,326¾	159,053½
Henry Goodwyn	62,885	545	
Edw. Burn. Green	33,753	1,032	82
William Green	4,440		3
Thomas Gutterſtone	1,018	3,907	
James Goddard	387	515	390
Mary Gwyn	105	104	700
Ann Groves	1½		93
H			
Peter Hammond	108,820		
George Hodgſon	19,099	532	57
John Hale	14,284	7,843½	10,453¼
George Hankin	12,385	206½	6,886
Thomas Holcombe	7,673	665	
Richard Harriſon	4,039	2,831½	9,471
John Hanbury	2,521	138	7,902
William Harding	3,273	1,532	261
Edmund Humphries	2,680		3,618
Thomas Hogsfleſh	2,556	1,748¼	1,357
George Healey	746	967	
James Holbrook	1,483		6,929
James Hogg	1,034	1,252½	
William Huxley	1,172	527	2,369
William Henſhaw	902		1,311
John-Robert Hawkins	473	241	1,091
Richard Hall	35		619
Howell Harris		1,281	575
James Harriſon			1,190
William Hoffman			1,163
Joſeph Harris		5¾	22
J			
Thomas Jordan	37,559	612	
James Johnſtone	2,320	1,256	6,585¼
John Johnſon	447	228	401
K			
Joſeph Kirkman	136	511	12,071
Thomas Kerſlake	54		1,300
John Krug	6	67	869
Carried over	868,227½	73,875¼	236,822¼

d 2   Brought

	Barrels of Strong	Barrels of Small	Barrels of Table Beer
L Brought over	868,227½	73,875¼	236,822¾
William Lancaster	33	28	3,799
Thomas Langford		564	1,101
M			
Richard Meux	57,520	1,014	
David Martineau	5,586	1,455	
John Rogers Morgan	6,493	398	8,820
James Myatt	1,400	124	655
Thomas Myatt	1,009	109	1,123
Mary Mercey	134		281
George Morcott	32¼		
Jane Moak			464
N			
William Newberry	12,653	619	
John Neiman	1,714	23	7,018
Henry Norgrove	34		834
O			
John Vaul Offner			1,207
P			
John Phillips, *Wapping*	49,558	531	
John Phillips, *Westminster*	7,570	663	67
Richard Parce	17,338		94
Thomas Proctor	16,862	351	
James Pulleine	5,060	813	1,787
Charles Page	5,751	1,641	395
James Purser	1,178	469	2,165
Richard Price	2,150	1,832¼	837¼
Joseph Pinnick	135		850
R			
William Truman Read	120,769	161	91
William Roberts	12,151	3,742	
James Robertson	2,555	500	1,327
Benjamin Ryall	906		2,107
John Robinson	11		1,140
John Robinson		1,076	2,462
Headman Raddatz	5	96	144
Carried over	1,196,835¼	90,085	275,590½ Brought

	Barrels of Strong	Barrels of Small	Barrels of Table Beer
S Brought over	1,196,835½	90,085	275,590¼
Robert Salmon ———	26,342	1,997	104
Thomas Stretton ———	11,524	107	6,816
Henry Sanford ———	2,604	———	19,467
Thomas Starkey ———	8,528	316	9,431
Benjamin Smith ———	1,544	———	4,504
William M. Sellon ———	5,039	59	3,981
William Simpson ———	4,600	3,358	3,725
Charles Shephard ———	4,735	189	6,447½
Seymour Stocker ———	2,159	1,888	———
John Stevens ———	180		214
William Shephard ———	398	———	4,553
James Stutter ———	68	———	688
George Stead ———	42	132	1,254
T			
Hester Lynch Thrale —	103,091	2,476	457
Thomas Taylor ———	158	———	564
Peter Thorne ———	43	———	55
V			
Thomas Vaughan ———	124	———	856
John Varty ———	70	———	1,382
W			
Samuel Whitbread ———	130,013	5,057	166
Joseph Williams ———	7,869	421	7,813
Samuel Watlington ———	2,211	1,329½	2,689
Crotchrode Whiffing ———	1,494	1,350½	1,760
Joseph Walker ———	756	———	2,917
Martin Willson ———	288	293	1,112
Thomas Whitehead ———	4,971	80	2,146
William Wilde ———	959	———	808
John Willson ———	176	———	4,942
James Willis ———	1,537	81	2,185
Robert Westmoreland —	567	1,671	432
Jos. Willmott ———	276	———	2,146
William Wright ———	———	———	3,189
Robert Walford ———	48	———	34
Y			
Benj. Yarnold ———	———	———	2,515
Total —	1,519,249½	110,890	374,943

CONTENTS.

CONTENTS.

Intro-

E R R A T A.

Page 32, line laſt, for *paler* read *pale.*
———, 52, line 21, dele *comma* after *art.*

*** Should any other errors occur in this volume, it is hoped the candor of the reader will excuſe the Author, whoſe attention to buſineſs of more immediate importance pievented him that careful reviſion which he ſhould otherwiſe have effected.

THEORETIC HINTS

O N

An Improved Practice

O F

BREWING MALT-LIQUORS;

Including fome Strictures

O N T H E

NATURE and PROPERTIES

O F

WATER, MALT, and HOPS;

The Doctrine of *Fermentation*;

The Agency of *Air*;

The Effects of *Heat* and *Cold*

On fermented Liquors, &c. &c.

Rerum cognofcere caufas.   VIRG.

The FOURTH EDITION, corrected.

PREFACE

TO THE

THEORETIC HINTS

O N

BREWING.

THE defign of the Author, in the publication of the fubfequent pages, is rather to intimate the probability of a *complete fyſtem of brewing*, than to promulgate one. Were he prompted by inclination to the undertaking, his intereſt would forbid the execution of it. The ordinary emoluments ariſing from the ſale of a book, however extenſive, would be a compenſation very inadequate to the fatigue of many years wearifome attention to the multifarious practice of a brewhouse, employed in the production of almost every species of malt-liquor; or to the trouble of digesting the œconomy of that practice, noting events, investigating causes, and thence forming rules for the regulation and management, of future processes. To the ingenious, it is presumed, these hints will not want utility, and to the mind unaccustomed to scientific disquisitions, a more perfect theory, without practical elucidation, might have been inefficacious. To both, in the present instance, the illustration of practice is necessary, where it is the intention of the enquirer perfectly to understand, in order to adopt, the principles upon which

the

the Author's fyftem is founded, to which this publication is defigned as preliminary, information only.

Such an illuftration muft be per-fonal, in confequence of fpecial agreement; from which it is prefumed that the brewery of London might vie with the country in the production of the finer *ales*, whilft the country brewer, in re-turn, might be convinced of the practicability of producing *porter* in his own office, of qualities equal, in every refpect, to thofe of the fame liquor brewed in the metro-polis. Locality, in either cafe, is no further concerned in peculiar qualities (climate only excepted) than what arifes from the difference

in

in the nature of the water, which being ſo large a portion of the pro-duct, has indeed a very powerful influence. Yet, by a knowledge of the cauſes of that influence, we are enabled to make an artificial variation of proceſs ſupply natural defect, and to prove that common, which was before thought to be peculiar.

From experimental practice in ſeveral different parts of the king-dom, the Author is convinced of this truth; nor is he leſs aſſured, from obſervations on the conti-nent, of the practicability of produ-cing malt-liquors in all the northern parts of Europe (except where the cold is ſo intenſe as to prevent the

action

action of fermentation) in as great perfection as in England. The climate of France, from Paris northward, of the French and Austrian Netherlands, of Holland, and of many parts of Germany, is well adapted to the brewing business, but the brewers know not how to reap the benefit of their situation. Those of Paris are entirely ignorant of the art, as well as that of malting. Their malts have but just time to germinate ere they are dried off, whence they have scarce any of the fermentable principles of a perfect malt in them, and are of so steely a consistence as to be hardly penetrable. Under these disadvantages, it is not to be wondered at that their *bonne*

bierre

bierre de Mars is fuch a miferable beverage. Did they purfue the method of malting inculcated in the following pages, and adopt a proper procefs of brewing, the fame quantity which they now make of wretched beer, for the retail price of fix fous the bottle, might be converted into a good porter, which fells there for 25 fous, or a pleafing pale ale of equal value. And tho' this increafe of price might not be entirely or immediately effected, on account of a prejudice common to all nations, of viewing in a fecondary light every imitation, however near the original, yet it is uncontrovertible that fuch a change in the quality, from a thin, ill-flavored, fpiritlefs, to a

pleafant,

pleafant, fprightly, vinous liquor, would be productive of emoluments exceeding, beyond all comparifon, the expence attending the acqui- fition ; and to confider it in a pub- lic light; it will occur to every per- fon, how much more wholefome and invigorating muft a found, nu- tritious malt-liquor be, than a mea- gre, hungry, ungenial wine, a liquor next in degree above the crude, un- formed beer here alluded to.

The Flemings, with every local advantage, are not many degrees beyond the French in the art of brewing, tho' malt-liquor is a be- verage much more common in Flanders than in France. At Bruf- fels, which fome writers have cele-

C   brated

brated for its beers, the beſt to be met with, in common, is of a browniſh amber, ſomewhat ſtrong and tranſparent, but, for want of being brewed by a ſkilful artiſt, it fails in point of preſervation, and turns acid in warm weather. They have another ſort, pale and turbid, called *bierre blanche de Louvaine*, which is little better than thick ſmall beer. This being bottled whilſt new, is no ſooner uncorked than it flies furiouſly out of the bottle, like beer in the height of fermentation, and is drunk by the Flemings in that ſtate, with much ſeeming reliſh, tho' they acknowledge, at the ſame time, that *it is not ſo good as Engliſh beer.*

The ſituation of Flanders is exceedingly favorable to the production

tion of malt-liquors, particularly in and about Bruffels. The foil is rich and fertile, well cultivated, and produces plenty of very good corn and hops, the latter of which are generally injured by hanging too long upon the plant, and by being gathered flovenly and bagged carelefsly. The air is very much like that of many parts of England, and there is a plentiful fupply of water, fit for every purpofe of the brewer. But the beneficence of Nature will be unavailing, fo long as her hand-maid, Art, withholds her neceffary aid. Were the Flemings to court the liberal difpenfation of her favors, and obtain a knowledge of the principles of brewing, they might foon difpute the palm with England in the celebrity of malt-liquors; for even here, the number of places entitled to any degree of pre-eminent diftinction is exceedingly limited, whilft the majority of practitioners do but barely overtop thofe of Flanders.

This extreme dearth of information, on a fubject of fuch general utility and importance, ought rather to be treated as a misfortune than a fault. Few, very few, of thofe employed in the practice of a brewhoufe, have ever been taught to confider brewing in any other than a mere mechanical light. Every mafter of a country ale-houfe, every hoftler of a country inn, every fervant of a country farmer, pretends

to

to a proficiency in the art, and the man of fcience is amazed to hear the common brewer dwell upon unaccountable difficulties, in a bufinefs practifed with feeming eafe, even by old women. Nor have thofe who have taken upon them to write particularly on the fubject, done any thing more than jumble together a number of recipes, in the ftyle and manner of a *cookery-book,* or *family phyfician,* but with fomewhat lefs efficacy. From thefe, one only may be excepted, who had the misfortune to be too abftrufely philofophical for common comprehenfion, and refined upon trifles till his theory frittered away the intention of his practice, and the product of both compleated their entire demolition.

The

The few ftrictures here fubmitted to the infpection of the public, are not brought forward as the refult of any deep refearches into the chymic art, but as the leading principles of an improved fyftem of brewing, founded, indeed, on the eftablifhed laws of chymiftry, but confirmed, in every reciprocal relation of caufes and effects, thro' a feries of practice of many years continuance.

Hence is the Author enabled to recommend, with confidence, his theory, as an illuftration of his practice; and his practice, as a confirmation of his theory; at the fame time that he propofes an appeal to well-attefted facts, as an additional ratification of both.

THEORETIC

THEORETIC HINTS

ON

BREWING.

Of WATER.

THE general diftinction of water, as it refpects the common purpofes of life, extends no further than the fimple terms of *hard* and *foft*; and tho' it may not be in the power of every brewer to purfue his inclination in the choice of them, yet as there are fome who can benefit of the diftinction, by the poffeffion of both, and as all may profit by the judicious application of either, it may not be amifs to fay fomewhat by way of diferiminating their virtues, and pointing out their ufes in brewing.

Hard water, is that which being ftrongly impregnated with certain terreftrial matters, does not eafily lather with foap, but

caufes

causes it to curdle or coagulate, and is in general less fit for culinary purposes. Its specific gravity is greater than that of soft water,* whence its power as a menstruum is proportionably lessened; but the experienced brewer, in some measure, guards against this inconvenience, by exposing his water, as much as he can, to the softening virtue of the air, and by varying the extracting heat, which in hard water produces effects at a certain degree, similar to those producible only at a distant degree in soft. This, however, has only relation to one species of malt-liquor; for with respect to the rest, the practice is unnecessary, if not prejudicial to the production of very desirable qualities.

In fermentation we find a considerable difference in the use of hard water, which does not at first so readily incline to that action, but it occasions a more violent, tho' less durable, operation than soft. As a preservative it may be preferred, on account

---

* Vide Appendix to *Statical Estimates.*

count, of its containing some alkaline
qualities, which contribute to counteract
any tendency to acidity in the beer, and
thence assist in its preservation. Tranfparency is, also, more easily obtainable
by the use of hard water; first, from its
inaptitude to extract such an abundance
of that light mucilaginous matter,
which, floating in the beer, for a long
time occasions its turbidity; secondly,
from its greater tendency to a state of quietude, after the vinous fermentation is
finished, by which those floating particles
are more at liberty to subside; and lastly,
from the mutual aggregation of the earthy
particles of the water with those of the
materials; which, by their greater specific
gravity, thus aggregated, not only precipitate themselves, but carry down also that
lighter mucilage just mentioned. For
these reasons it is not well adapted to the
brewing of porter, and such beers as require a fulness of palate, when drawn to
the great lengths of the London brewery,
and of some country situations. But we

D   can,

can, by a judicious application of the extracting heat, and a peculiar mode of conducting the action of fermentation, produce from hard water, as far as Art can
be the substitute of Nature, those qualities
which by unvaried practice are only obtainable from soft.

By *soft water* we mean that which being unburthened with the rigid earths, is
of less specific gravity, of more simple taste,
and of greater purity, which renders it
more capable of entering the pores, and
forming a solution of such parts of the
materials as yield to the impression of the
simple element.

The purity of water is determined by
its lightness, and in this distilled water,
only, can claim any material degree of perfection.   Rain water is the purest of all,
naturally produced; but by the perpetual
exhalation of vegetables, and other fine
substances floating in the atmosphere, it
does not come down to us entirely free of
those qualities which pond and river waters
possess in a greater degree.   These, especially

tially of rivers running thro' fens and morasses; from the quantity of grass and weeds growing therein, imbibe an abundance of vegetable solutions; which occasions them to contain more fermentable matter, and consequently to yield a greater portion of spirit; but at the same time induces such a tendency to acidity as will not easily be conquered. This is more to be apprehended towards the latter end of the summer; than at any other season of the year; because these vegetable substances are then in a state of decay, and thence more readily impart their pernicious qualities to the water which passes over them.

At such an unfavorable time should the brewer be necessitated to pursue his practice; it will behove him to pay the utmost attention to the cause of this disposition in his liquor; and thence endeavor to prevent the ill consequences, by conducting his process to the extraction and combination of such parts of the materials; as his judgment informs him will best counteract its effects.

D 2

Where

Where there is the liberty of choice,
I fhould recommend the ufe of that water which, from natural purity, equally
free of the aufterity of imbibed earths, and
the ranknefs of vegetable faturation, has a
foft fulnefs upon the palate, is totally fla-
vorlefs, inodorous, and colourlefs, whence
it is the better prepared for the reception
and retention of fuch qualities as the procefs of brewing is to communicate and
preferve.

Of MALT.

THE end of the procefs of malting
is well known, to every one concerned in the making and confumption of
malt, to be the production of that *faccharum*, upon which its value fo eminently depends ; but in the means of ac-
complifhing it, they are not fo entirely
agreed. In dry barley we find no appearance of this quality; the firft efforts of vegetation difcover none; let them continue

a

a little longer, and we perceive its gradual production to a certain period; beyond that period it again begins to disappear, and is soon totally lost.

To investigate the causes of these extraordinary changes, were a fruitless enquiry. Philosophy may amuse itself in tracing the imaginary gradation, till it be lost with the principle it pursues. The man of business will here find a better account in noting effects than in attempting to discover causes, which in the productions of Nature will ever be hypothetical, till Art can make the copy like the original.

In the business of malting, similar effects, in different subjects, are not produced at the same time, nor in the same apparent state of the grain, but vary according to their several natures and qualities. Thus Indian corn, and all the larger bodied grain is found to require a length of time sufficient to shoot out a considerable acrospire, before the production of its saccharine matter is perfect, whilst that of barley would be entirely destroyed by the same practice. The

The procefs of making malt is an artificial, or forced vegetation, in which the nearer we approach the footfteps of Nature, in her ordinary progrefs, the more certainly fhall we arrive at that perfection of which the fubject is capable. The farmer prefers a dry feafon to fow his corn in, that the common moifture of the earth may but gently infinuate itfelf into the pores of the grain, and thence gradually difpofe it for the reception of the future fhower, and the action of vegetation. The maltfter cannot proceed by fuch flow degrees, but makes an immerfion in water a fubftitute for the moifture of the earth, where a few hours infufion is equal to many days employed in the ordinary courfe of vegetation, and the corn is accordingly removed as foon as it appears fully faturated, left a folution, and confequently a deftruction of fome of its parts fhould be the effect of a longer continuance in water, inftead of that feparation, which is begun by this introduction of aqueous particles into the body of the grain.   Were

Were it to be fpread thin, after this removal, it would become dry, and no vegetation would enfue; but being thrown
into the couch, a kind of vegetative fermentation commences, which generates
heat, and produces the firft appearance of
germination. This ftate of the barley is
nearly the fame with that of many days
continuance in the earth, after fowing,
but being in fo large a body, it requires
occafionally to be turned over, and fpread
thinner; the former to give the outward
parts of the heap their fhare of the acquired warmth and moifture, both of which
are leffened by expofure to the air; the
latter to prevent the progrefs of the vegetative to the putrefactive fermentation,
which would be the confequence of fuffering it to proceed beyond a certain degree.

To fupply the moifture thus continually
decreafing by evaporation and confumption, an occafional, but fparing fprinkling
of water fhould be given to the floor, to
recruit the languifhing powers of vegetation,

tion, and imitate the shower upon the corn
field. But this should not be too often
repeated; for as in the field too much
rain and too little sun produce rank stems
and thin ears, so here would too much
water, and of course too little dry warmth,
accelerate the growth of the malt, so as to
occasion the extraction and loss of such of
its valuable parts, as by a slower process
would have been duly separated and left
behind.

By the slow mode of conducting vegetation here recommended, an actual and
minute separation of the parts takes place.
The germination of the radicles and acrospire carries off the cohesive properties of
the barley, thereby contributing to the
preparation of the saccharine matter,
which it has no tendency to extract, or
otherwise injure, but to increase and me-
liorate, so long as the acrospire is confined
within the husk; and by as much as it is
wanting of the end of the grain, by so
much does the malt fall short of perfection, and in proportion as it has advanced beyond, is that purpose defeated.

This

This is very evident to the moſt common obſervation, on examining a kernel
of malt, in the different ſtages of its progreſs. When the acroſpire has ſhot but
half the length of the grain, the lower
part, only, is converted into that mellow
ſaccharine flour we are ſolicitous of, whilſt
the other half exhibits no other ſigns of
it, than the whole kernel did at its firſt
germination. Let it advance to two-
thirds of the length, and the lower end
will not only have increaſed its ſaccharine
flavor, but will have proportionally extended its bulk, ſo as to have left only a
third part unmalted. This, or even leſs
than this, is contended for by many maltſters, as a ſufficient advance of the acroſpire, which they ſay has done its buſineſs
as ſoon as it has paſſed the middle of the
kernel. But we need ſeek no further for
their conviction of error, than the examination here alluded to.

Let the kernel be ſlit down the middle
and taſted at either end, whilſt green, or
let the effects of maſtication be tried, when

E   it

it is dried off; when the former will be
found to exhibit the appearances juſt
mentioned, the latter to diſcover the un-
wrought parts of the grain, in a body of
ſtony hardneſs, which has no other effect
in the maſh-tun than that of imbibing a
large portion of the liquor, and contributing to the retention of thoſe faccharine
parts of the malt which are in contact with
it; whence it is a rational inference, that
three buſhels of malt, imperfect in this
proportion, are but equal to two of that
which is carried to its utmoſt perfection.
By this is meant the fartheſt advance of
the acroſpire, when it is juſt burſting from
its confinement, before it has effected
its enlargement. The kernel is then uniform in its internal appearance, and of a
rich ſweetneſs in flavor, equal to any thing
we can conceive obtainable from imperfect vegetation.   If the acroſpire be ſuffered to proceed, the mealy ſubſtance melts
into a liquid ſweet, which ſoon paſſes into
the blade, and leaves the huſk entirely
exhauſted.

The

The fweet thus produced by the infant efforts of vegetation, and loft by its more powerful action, revives and makes a fecond appearance in the ftem, but is then too much difperfed and altered in its form, to anfwer any of the known purpofes of art.

The periods of its perfect appearance are, in both cafes, remarkably critical. It is at firft perfect at the inftant the kernel is going to fend forth the acrofpire, and form itfelf into the future blade; it is again difcovered perfect when the ear is laboring at its extrication, and haftening the production of the yet-unformed kernels. In this does it appear the medium principle of Nature's chymiftry, equally employed by her in her mutation of the kernel into the blade, and her formation thence of other kernels, by which fhe effects the completion of that circle to which the operations of the vegetable world are limited.

Were we to enquire, by what means the fame barley, with the fame treatment, produces unequal portions of the faccha-

rine

rine matter, in different fituations, we
fhould perhaps find it principally owing
to the different qualities of the water ufed
in malting. Hard water is very unfit for
every purpofe of vegetation, and foft will
vary its effects according to the predominating quality of its impregnations. Pure
elementary water is in itfelf fuppofed to
be only the vehicle of the nutriment of
plants, entering at the capillary tubes of
the roots, rifing into the body, and there
depofiting its acquired virtues, perfpiring
by innumerable fine pores at the furface,
and thence evaporating, by the pureft diftillation, into the open atmofphere, where
it begins anew its round of collecting
frefh properties, in order to its preparation for frefh fervice.

This theory leads us to the confideration of an attempt to increafe the natural
quantity of the faccharum of malt by adventitious means; but it muft be obferved, on this occafion, that no addition to
water will rife into the veffels of plants,
but fuch as will pafs the filter; the pores
of

of which appearing fomewhat fimilar to the fine ftrainers or abforbing veffels employed by Nature in her nicer operations, we by analogy conclude, that properties fo intimately blended with water as to pafs the one, will enter and unite with the economy of the other, and *vice verfa.*

Suppofing the malt to have attained its utmoft perfection, according to the criterion here inculcated, to prevent its farther progrefs, and fecure it in that ftate, we are to call in the affiftance of a heat fufficient to deftroy the action of vegetation, by evaporating every particle of water, and thence leaving it in a ftate of prefervation fit for the prefent or future purpofe of the brewer.

Thus having all its moifture extracted, and being, by the previous procefs, deprived of its cohefive property, the body of the grain is left a mere lump of flour, fo eafily divifible, that the hufk being taken off, a mark may be made with the kernel, as with a piece of foft chalk. The extractible qualities of this flour are, a fac-
.charum,

charum, clofely united with a large quantity of the farinaceous mucilage peculiar
to bread corn, and a fmall portion of oil,
enveloped by a fine earthy fubftance, the
whole readily yielding to the impreffion
of water, applied at different times and
different degrees of heat, and each part
predominating in proportion to the time
and manner of its application.

In the *curing* of malt, as nothing more
is requifite than a total extrication of every
aqueous particle, if we had, in the feafon
proper for malting, a folar heat fufficient
to produce perfect drynefs, it were practicable to produce beers nearly colorlefs;
but that being wanting, and the force of
cuftom having made it neceffary to give
our beers various tinctures and qualities
refulting from fire, for the accommodation
of various taftes, we are neceffitated to
apply fuch heats in the drying as fhall not
only anfwer the purpofe of prefervation,
but give the complexion and property
required.

To

To effect this, with certainty and precifion, the introduction of the thermometer is neceffary; but the real advantages
of its application are only to be known
from experiment, on account of the different conftruction of different kilns, the
irregularity of the heat in different parts of
the fame kiln, the depth of the malt, the
diftance of the bulb of the thermometer
from the floor, &c. &c. for tho' fimilar
heats will produce fimilar effects in the
fame fituation, yet is the difperfion of heat
in every kiln fo irregular, that the medium
fpot muft be found for the local fituation
of the thermometer, ere a ftandard can be
fixed for afcertaining effects upon the
whole. 'That done, the feveral degrees,
neceffary for the purpofes of porter, amber,
pale beers, &c. are eafily difcovered to the
utmoft exactnefs, and become the certain
rule of future practice.

Tho' cuftom has laid this arbitrary in-
junction on of variety in our malt-liquors, it
may not be amifs to intimate the loffes
we often fuftain, and the inconveniences
we

we combat, in our obedience to her man-
dates.

The further we purſue the deeper tints
of color, by an increaſe of heat beyond that
which ſimple preſervation requires, the
more we injure the valuable qualities of
the malt. It is well known that ſcorched
oils turn black, and that calcined ſugar
aſſumes the ſame complexion. Similar
effects are producible in malts, in proportion to the increaſe of heat, or the
time of their continuing expoſed to it.
The parts of the whole being ſo mutually
united by nature, an injury cannot be
done to the one without affecting the other;
accordingly we find, that ſuch parts of
the ſubject as might have been ſeverally
extracted, for the purpoſes of a more intimate union by fermentation, are, by
great heat in curing, burnt and blended ſo
effectually together, that all diſcrimination
is loſt, the unfermentable are extracted
with the fermentable, the integrant with
the conſtituent, to the very great loſs both
of ſpirituoſity and tranſparency. In paler
malts,

malts; the extracting liquor produces a feparation which cannot be effected in
brown, where the parts are fo incorporated, that unlefs the brewer be very well
acquainted with their feveral qualities and
attachments, he will bring over, with the
burnt mixture of faccharine and mucilaginous principles, fuch an abundance of
the fcorched oils as no fermentation can
attenuate, no precipitants remove; for
being in themfelves impediments to the
action of fermentation, they leffen its efficacy, and being of the fame fpecific gravity
with the beer, they remain fufpended in
and incorporated with the body of it, an
offence to the eye, and a naufea to the
palate, to the lateft period.

Of HOPS.

THE chymical principles of vegetables, as far as Art has yet been able
to difcover, by analyfis, are *water, falt,
oil,* and *earth.* Thefe, in different vegetables,

tables, do not only abound in different proportions, but vary in their fpecies and properties. The water, being only the general medium of the whole, is the fame fimple element in all; the oil in fome plants is more thin and fluid, in others more grofs and vifcous; the falt is in fome more volatile, in others more fixed; in fome acid, in others alkaline; the earth appears to be the mere uncharacteriftic refiduum of the whole, to which all have relation, and to which all finally return.

In hops, the quantity of oil is abun-dant; the finer part of an agreeable fra-grance and great volatility; the coarfer, from its intimate union with an auftere faline earth, of the alkaline kind, is groffer in its odour, harfher in its flavor, and lefs fubject to avolation.

The time of picking, the mode of curing, the care in bagging, the place of keeping, all have their fhare in the pre-fervation or deftruction of the finer qualities of this vegetable. If the hop be plucked too early, the confequence of im-maturity

maturity is obvious; if it hang too late,
the conftant avolation of its fine unctuous
parts, waftes its fragrance, deftroys its
color, and renders it of lefs value and efficacy. An application of too much heat
in the curing has fimilar effects; for by
evaporating the aqueous parts of the vegetable too haftily, the finer parts of the
effential oil rife with them and are loft,
whilft the remainder receives an injury
fomewhat fimilar to that of malt by the
like injudicious treatment. The care in
bagging and keeping is equally important, on the fame principle of excluding,
as much as poffible, the action of the external air upon the hop, which carries off
its more valuable qualities in the fame
manner as by a too long continuance on
the plant. The clofer they are preffed
down in the bag, the more effectual is
their fecurity againft this injury; and the
beft practical method of keeping them, is
in a clofe, but dry room, the bags laid upon each other, and the interftices well

filled

filled with a dry inodorous matter, fuch
as the firft fcreenings of malt, &c.

Time, however, will impair their virtues, in fpite of the utmoft precaution,
and that fo rapidly, as to render them incompetent to the nicer purpofes of the
pale-ale brewer, after the expiration of
the firft year, in all the ordinary modes
of preferving them.

In thefe virtues of the hop are we to look
for the primary principles of flavor and
prefervation of malt-liquors, which are to
be extracted in fuch manner and proportion, as to the judgment of the brewer
fhall feem moft likely to anfwer thofe intentions. To accomplifh this, with certainty and advantage, particular attention
muft be had to the feveral ends of extracting, and the different effects of thofe
extracts upon the reft of the procefs, viz.
whether the purpofe of flavor will not
defeat that of prefervation, and whether
the too anxious purfuit of prefervation
will not weaken the powers, and leffen the
effect of fermentation, to the very great
lofs

lofs of the fubject; for it is very certain, that every unctuous principle is an enemy to fermentation, and has a direct tendency to impair its action and deftroy its efficacy.

Hence are we taught by reafon, what is confirmed by experience, that the foluble parts of the hop, extracted feverally, an-fwer feveral different purpofes in beers, but taken collectively, tend to confound their virtues and pervert their ufes; and that in their extraction, if the means be not nicely proportioned to the end, the order of the procefs is deftroyed, and the intention of the brewer defeated.

Of WORTS.

HAVING taken a curfory view of the materials themfelves, we come now to confider more particularly the feveral modes of applying them, in order to extract their valuable parts, and the different effects of their application, in forming fuch extracts.

We

We have already feen that barley, by a partial vegetation, ftopped at a certain period, is converted into *malt*, a friable fub-ftance, eafily reducible to a mellow flour, the foluble principles of which are, a faccharum, very diftinguifhable by the fenfes, intimately united with a mealy, mucilaginous matter, and a fmall portion of oil enveloped by an earth.

The quality of the faccharine part refembles that of common fugar, to which it is practicable to reduce it, and its characteriftical properties are entirely owing to its intimate connection with the other parts of the malt, from which fuch diftinguifhing flavors of beers are derived, as are not the immediate refult of the hop. Were it not for thefe properties, the brewer might adopt the ufe of fugar, molaffes, honey, or the fweet of any vegetable, to equal advantage, which cannot now be done, unlefs an eligible fuccedaneum be found to anfwer that purpofe. As we are at prefent circumftanced, a fearch on the other fide would turn more to the brewer's account.

account. We have in malt a fuperabundance of the groffer principles, and would
government permit the introduction of a
foreign addition to the faccharine, which
is too deficient, many valuable improve-
ments might be made from it; as we
could, by a judicious application of fuch
adventitious principle, produce a fecond
and third wort of quality very little inferior to the firft.

But in thefe experiments, a very particular attention would be neceffary to the
folvent powers of the water at different
degrees of heat, and to the enquiry, How
far a menftruum already faturated with one
principle, may be capable of diffolving
another? Such a confideration is the more
neceffary on this occafion, to direct us
clear of two extremes equally difagreeable;
the firft is, that of applying the menftruum pure, and at fuch a heat as to bring
off an over proportion of the oleaginous
and earthy principles, which would occafion in the beer, thus wanting its fhare
of natural faccharum, a harfhnefs and aufterity,

fterity, which fcarce any time the brewer
could allow would be able to diffipate;
the other is, that of previoufly loading the
menftruum with the adopted fweet, in fuch
an abundance, as to deftroy its folvent
force upon the characteriftical qualities we
wifh to unite with it, and thereby leave it
a meer folution of fugar. The requifite
mean is that of confidering, what portion
of the faccharine quality has been extracted in the firft wort, according to the quantity of water and degree of heat applied,
and then to make fuch a previous addition
of artificial fweet as will juft ferve to coun-
terbalance the deficiency, and affimilate
with that portion of the remaining principles, we are taught to expect will be
extracted with the fucceeding wort.

From the nature of the conftituent
principles of malt, it is eafy to conceive
that the former, or faccharine and mucilaginous parts, yield moft readily to the
impreffion of water, and that at fo low a
degree of heat, as would have no vifible
effect upon the latter. If, therefore, we
                                    are

are to have a certain proportion of every part, it is a rational inference that the means of obtaining it refts in a judicious variation of the extracting heat, according to the feveral proportions required.

A low degree of heat, acting principally upon the faccharum, produces a wort replete with a rich, foft fweet, fully impregnated with its attendant mucilage, and in quantity much exceeding that obtainable from increafed heat ; which, by its more powerful infinuation into the body of the malt, acting upon all the parts together, extracts a confiderable portion of the oleaginous and earthy principles, but falls fhort in foftnefs, fullnefs, fweetnefs, and quantity. This is occafioned by the coagulating property of the mucilage, which, partaking of the nature of flour, has a tendency to run into pafte, in proportion to the increafe of heat applied, by which means it not only locks up a confiderable part of the faccharum contained therein, but retains with it a proportionate quantity of the extracting liquor, which would

G otherwife

otherwife have drawn out the imprifoned
fweet, thence leffening both the quantity
and quality of the worts.   And this has
fometimes been known to have had fo
powerful an effect, as to have occafioned
the *fetting of the goods*, or the uniting the
whole into a pafty mafs; for tho' heat
increafes the folvent powers of water, in
moft inftances, there are fome in which it
totally deftroys them.   Such is the prefent of flour, which it converts into pafte,
befides thofe of blood, eggs, and fome other
animal fubftances, which it invariably
tends to harden.

From a knowledge of thefe effects, we
form our firft ideas of the variations neceffary in the heat of the extracting liquor,
which are of more extenfive utility than
has been yet intimated, tho' exceedingly
limited in their extent, from one extreme
to the other.

The moft common effects of too low a
heat, befides fometimes producing immediate acidity, are an infipidity in the flavor
of the beer, from a deficiency of thofe characteriftical

racteriftical qualities before-mentioned;
and a want of early tranfparency, from
the fuperabundance of mucilaginous
matter, extracted by fuch heats, which,
after the utmoft efforts of fermentation,
will leave the beer turbid with fuch a
cloud of its lighter feculencies, as will
require the feparation and precipitation of
many months to difperfe.

The contrary application, of too much
heat, at the fame time that it leffens the
mucilage, has, as we have before feen, the
effect of diminifhing the faccharum alfo,
whence that lean, thin quality obfervable
in fome beers; and by extracting an over-
proportion of the oleaginous and earthy
principles, renders the bufinefs of fermentation difficult and precarious, and im-
preffes an aufterity on the flavor of the
liquor, which will not eafily be effaced.

Yet the true medium heat for each extract cannot be univerfally afcertained.
An attention not only to the quality of
the malt, but to the quantity wetted, is
abfolutely neceffary, to the obtaining every

due

due advantage; nor muft the period at which the beer is intended for ufe, be omitted in the account. The quality of the water, alfo, claims a fhare in the confideration, in order to fupply the want of folvent force in hard, and to allow for the natural lightnefs and fermentative quality of foft; a particular to which London, in a great meafure, owes the peculiar mucilaginous and nutritious quality of its malt-liquors; tho' it is not an improbable conjecture, that the water of the *Seine*, and of fome other large rivers, on the continent, would produce fimilar qualities by fimilar application.

Although the variations above alluded to are indifpenfible, it is eafy to conceive, from the fmall extent of the utmoft variety, that they cannot be far diftant; if, therefore, we know that a certain degree extracts the firft principles in a certain proportion, we need not much confideration to fix upon another degree that fhall produce the required proportion of
the

the remaining qualities, and effect that equal diftribution of parts in the extract, which it is the bufinefs of fermentation to form into a confiftent whole.

Of Boiling.

THE principal ufe of this operation, as it refpects the worts particularly, is to feparate the groffer or more palpable parts of the extract, preparatory to that more minute feparation which is to be effected in the gyle tun. The eye is a very competent judge of this effect; for the coagulations or concretions into which the continued action of boiling forms thofe parts, are obvious to the flighteft in-fpection, whilft the perfect tranfparency of the interftices of the worts, points out its utility in promoting that defirable quality in the beer.

In purfuing this obfervation, we have the fatisfaction to find the preceding
theory

theory of malt confirmed. The coagulating property of thefe parts, their fuperabundance in the firft wort, efpecially
from a low heat of liquor, the facility
with which they form, and the fuperior
bulk of the concretions in that wort,
fpeak them to be parts of that farinaceous
mucilage already explained; at the fame
time that the contrary appearances in the
fubfequent worts, their tardinefs to con-
crete, and the very minute particles into
which they form, in proportion to the
abundance of the oleaginous quality extracted with them, evince the nature and
exiftence of thofe other principles before
defcribed; for we find, by a common
culinary practice, that an unctuous and an
aqueous body may be fo intimately united,
by the interpofition of flour, and the action
of fire, as to become of a uniform confiftence; which being then diffufed in a
larger body of boiling water, the coagula-
tion of the flour, or the feparation of the
whole, would with greater difficulty be
produced than if fuch union had not been.
                                    With

With refpect to the utility of decoction in extracting the virtues of the hop, it may be necessary to recur to the consideration of that vegetable, in order to form some idea of the time requisite to the several intentions of extraction.

The fine effential oil of hops being most volatile and soonest extracted, we are thence taught the advantage of boiling the first wort no longer time than is sufficient to form the extract, without exposing it to the action of the fire so long as to dissipate the finer parts of this most valuable principle, and defeat the purpose of obtaining it. To the subsequent worts we can afford a larger allowance, and pursue the means of preservation so long as we can keep in view those of flavor, to which no rules can positively direct, the process varying with every variety of beer, and differing as effentially in the production of porter and that of pale ale, as the modes of producing wine and vinegar.

The confequence of not allowing a sufficient time for the due separation of the
parts

parts of the wort, and extraction of the
requisite qualities of the hop, is obvious
from what has been already said ; should
we proceed to the other extreme, we have
every thing to apprehend, from the introduction of too large a portion of the grosser
principles of the hop, which are very
inimical to fermentation, and from im-
pairing the fermentative quality of the
worts themselves, by suffering their too
long exposure to the action of the fire
passing thro' them, whereby they are reduced to a more dense consistence, and
their parts too intimately blended to yield
to the separating force of fermentation,
with that ease the perfection of the product requires.

Of Fermentation.

THE general definition of fermentation is, *a spontaneous internal motion of constituent parts, which occasions a
spontaneous*

spontaneous separation and removal from their former order of combination, and a remarkable alteration in the subject, by a new arrangement and re-union. This description is universal, and corresponds with the known effects of every species of the operation; but the particular kind to which our subject is limited, is the vegetable, which is again divided into the *vinous,* the *acetous,* and the *putrefactive,* forming a regular series or gradation, from the first origin of its action, to the total annihilation of the subject; or, as Dr. Shaw expresses it, "The intention or "tendency of Nature, is to proceed from "the very beginning of vinous fermen-"tation, directly, in one continued series, "to putrefaction, and thence again to a "new generation; which appears to be "the grand circle, wherein all natural "things are moved, and all the physical, "or rather chymical phænomena of the "globe produced."

It is not, however, the business of the artist to preserve this circle, but to break

H   the

the chain of connection in such parts as
may best answer the ends of his pursuit.
Thus, the brewer is to stop the progress of
the operation at the *vinous*, whilst the
vinegar-maker pursues it to the *acetous*,
beyond which every purpose of art is
defeated.

The result of vinous fermentation is
the production of that inflammable spirit,
which is no where to be found previous
to this action, and in which principally
the strength, or inebriating quality of
beers consists.   Hence it is evident, that
in proportion as we conduct fermentation
to that degree of perfection of which it is
capable, we shall produce that desirable
quality, and *vice versa.*

The only mode we are yet acquainted
with, of proving the presence of this spirit,
and determining the real strength of beers,
is by distillation, which is not only the
criterion of vinous fermentation, but the
proof of its perfection or imperfection,
by the quantity of spirit produced. By
the same means is the acetous fermentation

tion diftinguifhed, which fo alters, con-
ceals, or deftroys the inflammable fpirit,
that the ftill only throws over an acid,
uninflammable, aqueous liquor; which
feems to point out that regular progrefs
to the annihilation of the whole, which
putrefaction is to effect.

The principles produced by both thefe
fpecies of fermentation feem to be alike
purely *ethereal*; for they are fo exceedingly
volatile as to be in perpetual avolation, by
the common heat of the air only; but their
effects upon the human body are as widely
different as thofe of the operations which
produce them. That which refults from
vinous fermentation, being by the heat of
the ftomach thrown up into the head,
produces intoxication; whilft that from
the acetous, by a fimilar evaporation, in-
fenfibly pervades the veffels of the head,
and exfudes thro' the pores of the fkin,
with extreme fubtilty, in a vifible but cold
perfpiration. Thus are we taught to draw
the line of difcrimination in a feries of
caufes, from a knowledge of effects only;

or,

or, in other words, to determine the nature of the fermentation, from the quality of the principle produced.

The immediate fucceffion of the three fpecies feems to be the confequence of continuing the fubject in the fame ftate; for vinous fermentation is no fooner completed, than the acetous commences, if the fermenting liquor be fuffered to retain the fame degree of heat; in which ftate being incapable of depofiting its proper feculencies, their fufpenfion and commotion in the body of the liquor, continue the action beyond the period of vinofity, and the acetous fermentation of neceffity enfues; which by a fimilar continuation and expofure to the external air, would immediately produce the putrefactive, and proceed to the completion of that circle, in which all the labored combinations of Art, refolve into the firft fimple principles of Nature.

To mark the limits of diftinction, and ftop the progreffive force of fermentation, at fuch a period as fhall beft anfwer the

brewer's

brewer's purpofe, in the production of
every practicable degree of fpirituofity;
and to conduct the action to that period,
with every advantage to the fubject, is a
knowledge to be acquired not lefs from
practical attention, than theoretical enquiries. It is my bufinefs here, only to
affift the latter; the former requires an
elucidation fomewhat beyond the bounds
of verbal inftruction.

In the doctrine of fermentation, it is a
maxim, that *fuch fubjects as are moft fepa-*
rable by means of water, air, and heat,
have the greateft tendency to ferment; accordingly we find that wort, or the extract
of malt, abounds in fermentable matter,
but varies in quantity, in proportion to
the heat and quantity of the liquor employed, agreeable to our theory of extracts.
This fermentable matter we alfo find diftinguifhed into faccharine, mucilaginous,
oleaginous, and earthy. An adequate
proportion of each of thefe principles is
neceffary to a regular fermentation, and
the production of a perfect, uniform beer.

A

A furcharge of either, by deftroying the equilibrium, changes the mode of the action, difturbs the due arrangement of the parts, and produces effects agreeable to the nature of the predominating principle. Thefe effects, however, are not equally prejudicial to the beer; for we find that a furcharge of the faccharine and mucilaginous parts, tho' it occafions that turbidity and rawnefs of flavour before-mentioned, is yet corrigible by time, and yields very readily to the action of precipitants; but an over-proportion of the oleaginous and earthy principles, befides the evils before enumerated, efpecially from the browner malts, is frequently productive of two of the moft difagreeable qualities which ever difgraced the London brewery, where they have been particularly prevalent, and which time cannot correct, nor art effectually remove.

A due proportion of the fermentable principles being obtained, our next care is to collect the extracts into a body at fuch a degree of heat as will facilitate the action,

and

and to apply fuch a portion of a proper ferment, as fhall regulate and conduct it to the defired period of perfection.

It is well known that the juices or extracts of all faccharine vegetables, have a natural and fpontaneous tendency to ferment into a vinous liquor; this is alfo the property of wort, but the effects are not fimilar. The expreffed juices of fruits, the faccharine fap of certain trees, &c. when collected into a body at a due degree of heat, of themfelves produce a wine, without the addition of a ferment; but worts, being loaded with an abundance of a tenacious mucilage, without yeaft to affift and accelerate the efforts of nature, would run into an irregular and imperfect fermentation, or rather would immediately commence that *tumultuary motion* of their component parts, which is faid to produce putrefaction. This is, in a great meafure, confirmed by the effect; for tho' we find that the action has been fo far vinous as to produce a fmall portion of inflammable fpirit, yet the putrefactive has at the fame time

time been fo prevalent as to render the whole body of the liquor fetid and nauseous in the extreme; a confequence often derived from fuffering worts to remain too long, or in too large a body, without yeaft, efpecially in warm weather, when they have a greater propenfity to ferment in a body of a few inches deep, than they have in cold, at the depth of as many feet.

A proper application of yeaft prevents this accident, and difpofes the parts of the wort to that feparation and new arrangement, on which the perfection of the product depends.

The quantity of fermentable matter, already in action, thus conveyed into the body of the wort, affifts its fpontaneous aptitude to ferment, and a violent ftruggle immediately enfues. The air contained in the yeaft, being rarefied by the increafed warmth it meets with in the wort, begins to break from its confinement, and efcape at the furface, which is the firft perceptible fign of fermentation. In the rapid progrefs of its particles towards the top, a

smart

smart attrition and collision are occasioned,
between those particles, the body of the
wort they pass through, and the grosser
parts, which are, by their gravity, in con-
tra-direction. By this attrition the oleaginous parts of the subject are separated,
(a property which air is peculiarly allowed
to possess) and, being more subtile and
disposed to elasticity, would be carried off
with the air, were they not too intimately
connected with and enveloped by the
earthy, which are both too weighty to fly
off, and too much inclined to collect and
aggregate, by which means they at length,
with the grosser mucilage, subside to the
bottom, in the form of lees. But before
this can be effected, by their adherence to
the particles of air, to which they form a
vehicle, they are rapidly carried to the surface, where the air bursting from them,
the heavier fall down again towards the
bottom, whilst the lighter are supported,
by the continual efflux of air, till the suc-
cessive bursting of bubble after bubble lets
them down again into the liquor, and sup-

I   plies,

plies their place with frefh matter. In
their passage downwards, they are met by
other innumerable particles of air, in the
famerapid progrefs upwards, by which they
are again carried to the furface, there to be
left as before, till by repeated falling, col-
lition, and attrition, fome of the oleaginous
particles are effectually feparated from the
carthy, and united with the faccharine,
to which they have a natural tendency, as
is evinced by the ready incorporation of
common fugar and effential oils, by tri-
ture only, whence their mifcibility with
aqueous fubftances is effected.

This union is no fooner formed, than
the continuance of the action proceeds to
abforb the finer parts of the earthy principle, which is left floating up and down
in the liquor, after its feparation from
the oleaginous ; by which addition, and
the intervention of the mucilage, that common medium, which fermentation rather
tends to refine than difunite, the whole is
converted into a compact and uniform
body.

The

The groffer parts having, by this violent commotion, been completely feparated, and the finer recompofed, the more weighty of the former fall to the bottom, whilft the lighter, confifting principally of the refufe mucilage, are carried to the top, where, by their glutinous adherence to each other, being fupported by the collected air, they form a yeafty head.

The action now languifhes, the vinous fermentation is complete, and all that is wanting, is the prevention of the further progrefs of the operation, by dividing the fubject into cafks, where it foon becomes of lefs heat, by which means the heavier particles condenfe and effectually fubfide; the lighter, by the frequent filling up of the cafks, are collected nearly to a point, at the bung-hole, where being thrown off, they fall down the fide, and leave the beer completely purged of all matter which might hereafter endanger a pernicious *ftubbornefs*, or deftructive *fret*.

Were a confirmation of this doctrine neceffary, we might perhaps find it in an

I 2 attentive

attentive obfervance of the effects of fermentation, at different periods or its action. That the oleaginous and earthy principles are firft ftruck out of the body of the wort, is evinced by its remarkably fweet flavor at that time, and the very grofs, bitter aufterity of the frothy head, which then contains the greater part of the unattenuated oils and earths; and that thofe principles do unite and incorporate with the faccharine and mucilaginous, in the latter part of the operation, is proved by the gradual alteration in the flavor of the liquor, from a mixed fweet to a uniform vinofity, and a fimilar change in the harfhnefs of the yeafty head, which then affumes a like uniformity, fo far as the term may be allowed to the aggregated refufe of fo many different principles.

The agency of air, in the bufinefs of fermentation, is very powerful, but as all fermentable fubjects have an abundant fupply, we are rather to provide for the egrefs of their own, than to fuffer the admiffion of the external air, by which a

great

great number of the fine, volatile, oleaginous parts of the fubject would be carried
off, and a proportionate injury in flavor
and fpirituofity fuftained. Hence fuch a covering fhould be provided for the gyle-tun
as would barely allow the efcape of the
common air produced by the operation,
whilft the *gas*, or fixed air, from its greater
denfity, refting upon the furface of the
beer the whole depth of the curb, prevents the action of the external air, and
confequently the efcape of thofe fine and
valuable parts juft mentioned.

This probable confequence is the more
to be depended on, from the known fimi-
larity of effect which gas produces upon
flame, which it immediately extinguifhes,
by preventing that rapid avolation of unctuous particles which is faid to conftitute
flame. In this inftance the external air
is the agent, which caufes and conducts
the avolation, and without a continual
fupply of which it cannot exift; this fupply being effectually cut off by an immerfion of the fubject in the gas of fermenting
liquor,

liquor, the flame is inftantaneoufly extin-
guifhed; nor will glowing fire itfelf exift
in it a long time, tho' it contributes to
rarefy and difperfe it; and to animals in-
haling it, a death as fudden as by a ftroke
of lightning is the confequence.

But towards the conclufion of vinous
fermentation, this aerial covering begins
to lofe its efficacy, which points out the
neceffity of then getting the beer into
cafks, as foon as poffible, that the confequences may be prevented, of expofing fo
large a furface, liable to fo copious an evaporation. Amongft thefe, a lofs of fpirituofity is not the leaft; for this evaporation
is more and more fpirituous, as the action
approaches the completion of vinous fermentation, and that once obtained, the
lofs becomes ftill more confiderable, if ftill
expofed to the air; whence it might be
termed the diftillation of Nature, in which
fhe is fo much fuperior to Art, that the
ethereal fpirit rifes pure and unmixed,
whilft the higheft rectification of the ftill
produces,

produces, at beſt, but a compound of aqueous and ſpirituous parts.

Nor is this entirely conjecture. Experience teaches us, that we cannot produce ſo ſtrong a beer in ſummer, *ceteris paribus,* as in winter; the reaſon is, not becauſe the action of fermentation does not realize ſo much ſpirit in warm weather, but becauſe the fermenting liquor, after the perfection of vinoſity, continues ſo long in a ſtate of rarefaction, that the ſpirituous parts are diſſipated in a much greater degree at that time, than at any other, in a ſimilar ſtate of progreſſion. And this doctrine of natural diſtillation ſeems to account for that increaſe of ſtrength obtainable from long preſervation*, in well-cloſed caſks, and, more particularly ſo, in glaſs bottles; for Nature, in her efforts to bring about her grand purpoſe of reſolving every compound into its firſt principles, keeps up a perpetual internal ſtruggle, as well as an external evaporation; and if the latter be effectually prevented, the former muſt be productive of additional ſpirituoſity,

* Vide *Statical Eſtimates,* &c.

tuofity, fo long as the action keeps within the pale of vinous fermentation.

In order to maintain a due regulation of the fermenting power, and to anfwer the feveral purpoſes of the operation, a fcrupulous attention to the degree of heat at which the action commences, and a particular regard to the quality and quantity of the ferment employed, are indifpenſibly neceſſary.

The quality of the yeaſt requires the more minute fcrunity, becauſe it is not poſſible to produce a perfect and effectual fermentation, without it be good, evinced by its lively, elaſtic appearance, and powerful effect in application. The quantity can only be aſcertained by the intention of the artiſt. In many inſtances, a larger portion is tantamount to a higher degree of fermenting heat, and *vice verſa* ; but this is chiefly confined to the purpoſe of accelerating the proceſs. If the operation be too languid, from a want of heat in the fermenting liquor, an addition of freſh yeaſt may fupply the deficiency, and effect

the

the required recompofition of parts, without which there is not only an immediate
lofs of ftrength, but fuch a derangement
of the prefervative principles, as will effectually prevent their re-union, and leave
the imperfect product to the certainty of
early deftruction. The action, in this
inftance, having only fufficient force to
feparate, and being unable to attenuate
and recompofe the oleaginous and earthy
parts of the fubject, the body of the beer
remains a heavy, unconcocted farrago of
the whole conftituent principles, of a ful-
fome, fweet, mawkifh flavor, prompt to a
ftubborn fret, on the firft change of air,
and confequent acidity, the final period of
its exiftence as a vinous liquor.

This, alfo, leads us to the neceffity of
completing the vinous fermentation, previous to *cleanfing*, or putting the liquor
into cafks, which change of quantity and
fituation alters the action from fermentation to *purgation* only ; for thofe parts
which in the gyle-tun are carried to the
top, and repeatedly fall again into the body

K of

òf the liquor, to be there further separated, attenuated, refined, and recompofed,
are, in the cafk, thrown off entirely, and
perifh in the *ftillion*, or receiver, before
they can be returned again, by filling up
the veffel.

The confequences of fuch a violent dif-
union, have been before noted; to which
may be added, the great lofs of fpirituofity,
occafioned by fo premature a divifion of
the fermenting liquor into fmaller quantities, which immediately checks the operation, and prevents its being brought to
a proper crifis, both from the preternatural
difcharge of the cafk, and the want of a
fufficient body to accomplifh that end;
for it is not in the power of art to produce a proportionate quantity of fpirit
from a fmall body of wort, to that which
is obtainable from a large one, tho' of
equal quality in every refpect.

The effects of a contrary conduct, in
fuffering the liquor to remain in the tun
after the period of vinous fermentation,
have been already fufficiently intimated;
but

but the criterion which marks the exact period of maturity, resting more upon the discrimination of the senses, than an appeal to the understanding, we must leave to the illustration of practice, what lies beyond the documents of theory to define.

In these strictures, the *use of the thermometer* has been all along implied, without which all theory is ineffectual, all practice uncertain. We have seen that the variation of a few degrees of heat in forming the extracts, produces an important difference of effect. In the heat of fermentation, similar consequences result from similar variety. Under a certain regulation of the process, we can retain in the beer, as far as art is capable, the finer mucilage, and thereby preserve that fullness upon the palate which is by many so much admired; on the other hand, by a flight alteration, we can throw it off, and produce that evenness and uniformity of flavor, which has scarce any characteristical property, and is preferred by some, only for the want of that heaviness which

they

they complain of in full beers. If a more vinous, racy *ale* be required, we can, by collecting and confining the operation within the body of the wort, cause the separation and abforption of fuch an abundant portion of the oleaginous and earthy principles, as to produce a liquor in a ftate of perfection at the earlieft period, and fo highly flavorous, as to create a fufpicion of an adventitious quality.

Thus, by a judicious management of this moft difficult and interefting part of the brewing procefs, we are enabled to influence natural flavor, fpirituofity, and prefervation. By a further improvement, we can introduce foreign virtues, (as in the inftance of *porter,* &c.) anticipate age, and produce in two months the properties and characterifticks of twelve.

Of Cellarage.

THE *diforders of the cellar* are frequently mentioned among the grievances of the brewer, tho' they have in

reality

reality no exiſtence. Every diſorder in beers has its origin in the brewhouſe, except thoſe which ariſe from palpable neglect; ſuch as the flatneſs occaſioned by leaving the veſſels unſtopped, and the conſequences ariſing from the uſe of a cellar ſo ill defended from the external air, as to expoſe the beer to every viciſſitude of weather, from the extremity of ſummer's heat, down to the ſeverity of winter's cold.

The former points out its own prevention, but its remedy muſt be ſought in a freſh fermentation, artfully introduced, and moderately conducted. Upon the latter, as a particular often diſregarded, a few thoughts may not be uſeleſs.

The temperature of the air to which beers ought generally to be expoſed, for the purpoſes of perfect preſervation, and the advantages of age, is that which equally avoids the two extremes, and is kept as uniformly invariable as the excluſion of either will permit. By Fahrenheit's thermometer we find the ſummer heat to be at 76 degrees, and the point of freezing

at

at 32. Experience teaches us to adopt the intermedium, as the moſt certain means of avoiding the effects of that rarefaction and natural diſtillation before treated of, and the contrary conſequences of advancing towards the oppoſite extreme of *concentration,* or freezing the aqueous parts of the liquor.

In proportion to the warmth of the air, as has been already intimated, the whole body is rarefied, the ſpirituous parts are thence more eaſily ſet at liberty, and their conſtant avolation increaſed ; by which a proportionate injury to the flavor, and a diminution of the ſtrength are effected ; for tho' the caſks may be very well cloſed, the extreme ſubtilty of this ſpirituous evapɒration will find means to pervade the head of the veſſel, which in a warm, dry ſituation, is not a little diſpoſed to favor the eſcape, whereas the humidity inſeparable from a cloſe, cool cellar, ſo ſaturates the wood as to render it, in a conſiderable degree, impervious to the flying vapor. Nor is this diſſipation of ſpirituous parts
thro'

thro' the pores of the wood, to be deemed the chimera of conjecture. We have a confirmation in point, in the known effect of keeping diftilled liquors in cafks, which is an evident lofs of ftrength, eafily demonftrable by the hydrometer or hydroftatic balance; whilft thofe kept in glafs, continue for years without any material alteration. But glafs itfelf is infufficient for the purpofes of the prefent occafion; becaufe the increafed heat of air excites a frefh commotion in the beer, which immediately proceeds to acidity, and the confequent mutation of the fpirit, from an inflammable to an uninflammable principle.

On the contrary, a degree of cold, as it approaches to the freezing point, by condenfing, proportionally leffens that difpofition to evaporate, but equally tends to concentrate the fpirituous parts; which would actually happen, fhould the degree of cold be fo intenfe as to freeze the liquor. In that cafe, the cold acts only upon the aqueous parts, beginning with thofe in

contact

contact with the veffel, and thence advancing towards the centre, forcing the fpirituous parts inwards, till the concentrated
liquor is of fufficient ftrength to refift an
extreme degree of cold, as has frequently
been inftanced in the freezing of a cafk of
fmall beer, in the manner here treated of,
to fuch a degree, that the liquor in the centre became of a quality equal to ftrong.

This is only quoted in order to intimate the difadvantages of concentration,
and, of courfe, all approaches thereto;
for the aqueous parts being, by that means,
gradually detached, become in a certain
degree pure water; and it is notorious that
water mixed with ftrong beer, as an occafional beverage, makes a difagreeable, flat,
double-flavored liquor. The effect of concentration, if not equal, is fimilar, as
would be experienced on the firft change
of air of fufficient warmth to fet thefe
aqueous or perifhed parts at liberty to re-
unite with the concentrated liquor; and
tho' this accident could fcarce ever happen
to a perfon but moderately attentive to his
businefs,

bufinefs, there are fome who approach too near the caufe of it, to be entirely un‑affected by the confequence.

Of the two extremes, an inclination to the latter may be leaft prejudicial, as only tending to a feparation, which it is in the power of a new fermentation to rectify, whilft the effects of the former are, a dif‑fipation of the more valuable parts, and a difpofition of the remainder to inevitable deftruction.

To purfue this fubject beyond its pre‑fent limits were to exceed the purpofe of the author, who referves the further elu‑cidation of his theory for the perfonal ap‑plication of thofe who may wifh to be more fully informed, by the convincing arguments of practical confirmation, and the corroborating teftimony of facts.

L   STATICAL

STATICAL ESTIMATES

OF THE

MATERIALS FOR BREWING;

OR,

A TREATISE on the APPLICATION and USE of

The SACCHAROMETER,

An INSTRUMENT conſtructed for the PURPOSES

Of regulating to ADVANTAGE

The OECONOMY OF THE BREWHOUSE,

And of eſtabliſhing the MEANS of producing

UNIFORM STRENGTH in MALT-LIQUORS;

Including a definite Eſtimate of the intrinſic Value of different MALTS, the Produce of ENGLISH, SCOTCH, and FOREIGN BARLEY; the ſpecific Gravities of WORTS, from which ſeveral Kinds of ALE and PORTER are made; the ATTENUATION of the DENSITY of fermentable Fluids, by the Action of Fermentation; the Portion of SPIRIT generated by that Action, in Beers of different Lengths; the Mode of eſtimating the STRENGTH or INEBRIATING QUALITY of fermented Liquors; with ſome Propoſitions for effecting a very conſiderable Saving in the Conſumption of MALT.

THE SECOND EDITION, REVISED AND CORRECTED.

By J. RICHARDSON.

Docet " ratione, modoque." HOR.

PREFACE

STATICAL ESTIMATES

Of the MATERIALS for BREWING.

SEVEN years * have elapſed ſince the
author of the following ſheets ad-
dreſſed himſelf to the public, on a ſubject
which, if at that time it attracted their
notice, will, it is conceived, as now pre-
ſented to them, be found to have ſtill a
greater claim to their attention. His
views, on that occaſion, were to effect an
eventual profit to the brewer, from the
melioration of his produce; on the
preſent, they are directed to his actual
and immediate advantage, from a reduction in the quantity of the materials
he employs.

The favourable reception which attended that addreſs, the ſucceſs reſulting

from

* The *Theoretic Hints on Brewing* were firſt pub-
liſhed in 1777, and the firſt edition of this Treatiſe in 1784.

from the practice it referred to, in the in-creased and increasing trade of those to whom it was communicated*, and their ingenuous and repeated acknowledgments of the advantages derived from it, have long been matter of pleasing reflection to him.

Incited by this to pursue his investiga-tions, he was determined to persevere till he should be able, if practicable, to rescue from the hands of ignorance and illiterature, the conduct of a business of such magnitude as the brewery of these kingdoms; and to give the features, form, and proportion of science to an object so highly valuable, which has been, for centuries past, disguised by obstinate stu-pidity, and deformed by the empiricism of ridiculous old women.

How

---

* The author still continues to communicate this practice, comprising the several processes of brewing *porter* and *pale malt-liquors*, of every species, the terms of which may be known by applying to him.

How far he has fucceeded in that attempt, on the prefent occafion, muft be
left to the candor of the impartial reader
to determine; and whether the end will
ever be entirely accomplifhed, is matter
of doubt. A fingle glance upon the diverfity of habits and fentiments of men in
general, will readily fuggeft obftacles
which ftand like mountains in the way.
New doctrines do not foon become objects of general affent; and the eftablifhment of a formal fyftem, where public
opinion has long denied the exiftence of
principles, is a work of no ordinary difficulty. The ingenuity of a Harvey firft
traced the vital current in our veins, but
it was unequal to the tafk of conquering
that habitual ftupidity which ftamped in-
credibility on the difcovery.

The humble origin of the brewing bufinefs has long entailed a general concur-
rent opinion, that its profeffors need
neither genius nor education; and in
conformity to that opinion, has this profeffion,

feffion, more, perhaps, than any other, of the like national importance, been difgraced by finking into the hands of the moft ignorant and illiterate; from whofe contracted underftandings, biaffed by the influence of ftrong prejudice, and rendered obftinate by the pride of long practice, the man who offers the adoption of a new fyftem, however clearly fupported by reafon, has a hoft of enemies to encounter *.

It is, however, a happinefs that the extenfive connections of modern times have induced

* If the reader be in the humour of fmiling at a proof of this obfervation, he may amufe himfelf for a moment, with the perufal of the following fpecimen of the *fcience* and *literature* of a country brewer, in Lincolnfhire, copied *verbatim & literatim* from his letter, which the author received in confequence of having put him to the important expence of *four pence,* for the poftage of his *Advertifement to the Brewers,* circulated in 1777. It contained the faid advertifement inclofed, in order to double the poftage, and is not the only epiftle of the kind with which the author was amufed at that time.

(COPY)

induced men of fortune, education, and liberality, in this country at leaſt, to adopt

(C O P Y.)

Sr,

I know Not who or what you are or what Profitchion you are off I have Recd, a long Rodda mantade about Nothing you have ſaid Nothing though there is a grate deal in your Paper you Point me to nothing how I am to avoid theſe actldents that may hapen So upon the whole I looke on it as a peſe of quackere you want to hum the Contre at any Rate if you can but Get there Caſh but I Defie you to Gard againſt what you Make Mention off I think My 45 years Expereance is a Match for your *there* Pray Sr, what would you have thaught of me if I had Sent you Such an apittle about My 45 years Expereance and Say as much upon it as you have dun on your *there* as not knowing me you would have thaught me A Sawfe Imperdent fellow to take upon me to Dictate to you about your Buiſneſs Put you to Charges and order to Poſt Pay yours to Me what rite have you to Dow this to me I ſay you are a Safe Imperdent fellow, whome Soever you are I thaught I Could not Make you a better Preſant then to ſend you your own a gaine, you are Sum Poor Roge or other or youd, never take Such lebertys to rit to Peopele you know Nothing off

To Mr. John Richatdſon Joe, Coffee Houſe
Mitre Fleet Street

M

adopt the profeffion, and render it refpectable. To thefe the author wifhes
more particularly to addrefs himfelf, in
the expectation that, influenced by their
example, others of a lefs fpeculative or
lefs comprehenfive turn of mind, may be
induced to try if they cannot difcover
fome fcientific *traits* in the objects of
their daily purfuits, and benefit themfelves
by the difcovery.

The introduction of the thermometer
into the practice of the brewery, general
as it is now becoming, was by flow
and cautious fteps. The fturdy ignorance
of a country fellow, dignified by the appellation of *brewer*, too often oppofed itfelf to the good fenfe and difcernment of
his employer, to the defeat of the intended
improvement; though it did not always
happen that this ignorance was unmixed
with *cunning*. There was fometimes an
apprehenfion that the inftrument might
become a rule in the mafter's hand, by
which the abilities of the fervant might
be meafured; and that the interference

of

of the former might prove deſtructive of the importance of the latter.

The prevalent practice of thoſe days (and it is not yet annihilated) was either to mix a given quantity of cold, to a given quantity of boiling water, in the copper, for the purpoſe of maſhing; or to turn the boiling water into the maſh-tun, and ſuffer it to remain till the brewer could *ſee his face in it*, before the malt was put into it; both of which are ſufficiently ridiculous to be diſcontinued, where the means of meaſuring heat are to be obtained. As an appendage to this practice, the finger ſupplied the place of a thermometer, in determining the fermenting heat of the wort, and the brewer was perſuaded that the delicacy of his ſenſations, in that buſineſs, precluded the neceſſity, and rendered impertinent the adoption of a ſubſtitute.

Some of the brewers on the continent carry the matter ſtill further, and determine the heat of the ſcalding liquor in-

tended

tended for mashing, by the finger also *.
One of these, to whom the author mentioned the use of the thermometer, in afcertaining the degrees of heat, replied,
with a significant nod of the head, attended with a kind of contemptuous smile,
*Monsieur, je sais la chaleur de l' eau par le
doigt, auffi bien que vous la savez par votre
instrument.*

So little, indeed, do the generality of
inferior brewers expect matter of science
in their business (though they frequently
affect great *secrecy)* that their inattention
to some circumstances, which force themfelves on their notice, is really a state of
warfare against common sense.

A

* Since the first publication of these remarks,
the author has been credibly informed, that the first
rudiments of the professional education of the
greatest brewer in this kingdom, were founded on
the principle here adduced. His hand was directed to be immersed in the liquor, and then to
make a short revolution in it. If he could bear only
one or two of these revolutions, the liquor was too
hot; but if he could just accomplish *three,* it was
in a proper state for mashing.

A gentleman of veracity affirms, that having obferved to a brewer of this character, that his under-back was *leaky*, and that he was fubject to a daily lofs in the quantity of wort wafted thereby; the other exclaimed " Not at all l I lofe no" thing by the little wort which runs out, " for *I always draw my ufual length.*" In other words, he made up with water what he loft in wort, and fo thought himfelf no fufferer. It is much to be feared, that upon fuch an œconomift, the doctrines hereafter inculcated will have little influence.

It frequently happens, too, that men of plain good fenfe, from not being accuftomed to think abftrufely, or to turn their minds to fcientific fubjects, do conceive moft extravagant ideas, when a thought relative to thefe matters happens to ftrike their imagination. A very refpectable perfon of this defcription, fpeaking of the gravity of wort, alledged, that the variation of that circumftance could be no certain foundation for variety of ftrength

in

in the beer; " becaufe, faid he, I could
" add to its gravity by putting falt into it;
" or I could make a mixture of falt and
" water of the fame gravity, and yet the
" wort with the falt in it would not be
" productive of an increafe of fpirit pro-
" portioned to its increafed gravity, and
" the falt and water would produce none."
In the fame manner it might be infifted,
that the fuperior lightnefs of a fpirituous
fluid is no proof of fuperior ftrength, becaufe it is in the power of a perfon to
dulcify the ftrongeft fpirit, till it is as
heavy as the weakeft, that it may elude
the detection of every ftatical apparatus.

On the other hand, there are thofe who,
from a conviction of the inefficacy of the
common modes of eftimating the value
of malt, are induced to rack their invention with the view of arriving at a
more certain determination, though the
means they adopt often prove as inadequate as thofe they have rejected. Amongft
thefe may be reckoned the attempt of an
old gentleman in the north-weft of England,

land, who, after having mafhed a fmall
quantity of malt in a tea-pot, held a
grand convocation, confifting of himfelf,
his wife, and his moft experienced fer-
vants, who, in due form, fat in judgment upon its merits, which were to be
determined by the evidence of the palate,
in tafting the wort; when, after due
difcuffion, the decifion of the majority
was agreed to be final, and the malt was
valued accordingly. This curious circumftance the old gentleman related, with
great good humour, on feeing the author's
apparatus hereafter defcribed, thereby intimating a juft fenfe of the want of fuch
certain means of difcriminating the value
of the materials, and a ready docility to
adopt them whenever they fhould be obtainable.

The darknefs in which the bufinefs of
brewing is involved, extends even to the
legiflature itfelf, as is evinced by the frequent difputes between brewers and officers of excife, on the fubject of diftinguifhing worts chargeable with the ftrong beer
duty,

duty, from thofe which are to be charged only as fmall; and this feems to have oc-cafioned the late act of parliament, for ma-king a feparate and advanced charge upon *table beer*, to be compulfatory upon the brewer *to brew it alone*; that the officer may not be puzzled in applying his only means of difcrimination, confifting in dipping his finger into the wort, tafting it, &c. and from thefe inftances it may be perceived, that the finger is or has been a very important agent both to the brewer and the revenue officer, in the exercife of their different functions. In this ignorance, alfo, originate thofe ridi-culous reftrictions which prohibit the mixing of fmall with ftrong beer, in order to accommodate the palate of any perfon with the liquor he prefers. Were the duties charged according to the fpecific gravity of the wort, thefe altercations would immediately vanifh, the revenue would be increafed, the brewer would be at liberty to make, alter, or compound his liquor into as many and as various

forts,

forts, as he has palates to pleafe, without fubjecting himfelf to the interference of the officer, or the lafh of the law.

As it is not, however, the bufinefs of the author to prefcribe legiflative regulations, he has only to affert, that from a long experience of the utility and beneficial efficacy of the inftrument hereby offered to the attention of the public, he has the cleareft conviction of the accuracy with which it accomplifhes the purpofe intended by the whimfical effay above quoted, and of the great advantages derivable to the brewery from its general adoption, even were its ordinary application, only, as directed and explained in the treatife, to be the object of that adoption ; but fhould the extraordinary practice, difcovered in the courfe of his experiments, and propofed, in the *poftfcript*, to be particularly communicated, become alfo an univerfal practice with every brewer, the event, exclufive of the former confideration, muft be a confiderable reduction in the general price of the mate-

N　　　　　rials,

rials, as well as a particular faving to individuals, in the quantity confumed.

To particularife its effects on the price
of malt, o ly, as the article from which
the greateft advan.age is to be derived,
it needs only to be confidered, that if the
mo.t moderate computation of the average
faving, refulting from the extraordinary
practice above alluded to, be *five per cent.*
in the general confumption, the event of
that diminution would be equivalent to
an increafe in the natural product of the
earth to that amount; for if the then
annual confumption of malt be fignified
by 95, and there be 100 brought to market, the fupply exceeding the demand,
in that proportion, muft of neceffity produce a proportionate reduction in the
price.   Hence a double advantage would
accrue to the brewer; firft, from the general event, which leffens the price; and
then from his particular faving in quantity, calculated at the reduced rate.

Let us fuppofe, for the fake of ftating
the matter clearly, that a perfon brews at
one

one time thirty quarters of malt, for which, as things are now circumstanced, he pays forty shillings per quarter, making the whole cost sixty pounds. Let us then suppose the improvement alluded to has taken place generally, so as to have reduced the price in a ratio of two shillings per quarter; in which case the same person, adopting the improved practice, and brewing the same quantity of liquor, of the same specific strength, would find himself thus advantageously situated.

Instead of 30 quarters of malt, which at 40 s. per quarter would cost — £ 60 0 0
Deducting the five per cent. saving, he would only use 28¹ quarters at 38 s. £ 54 3 0

Whence the difference in favour of the above practice is — — — — — £ 5 17 0

This, at first sight, appears a clear gain of 10 *per cent.* but, on a further examination, it will be found to exceed that proportion.

If we suppose the present annual consumption of such a brewer to be 3000 quarters of malt, and that its cost is £6000; then making a deduction of 150

quarters

quarters from the quantity confumed, for the fuppofed faving of five per cent. and of 2 s. per quarter from the price, for the fuppofed general reduction, in confequence of a general adoption of the practice recommended, the fimple advantage attainable thereby, in this inftance, may be thus calculated :

State of the prefent practice.

Capital required for 3000 quarters of
 malt, at 40 s. — — — — £ 6000 0 0
One year's intereft on the fame — —   300 0 0

       Total £ 6300 0 0

State of the propofed improvement.

Capital required for 2850 quarters of
 malt, at 38 s. five per cent. being
 deducted from the quantity and price,
 as above eftimated — — — £ 5415 0 0
One year's intereft on the fame — 270 15 0

     Total £ 5685 15 0
Annual faving by this plan — — 614 5 0

      £ 6300 0 0

        Hence

Hence it is evident that there would be a net *additional* profit of near *eleven per cent.* on the £5415 advanced, besides the convenience of making that sum supply the place of £6000, effecting thereby a reduction of capital to the amount of near ten per cent. which is an object of no small importance, where money is not abundant.

As the probable means of universal benefit, this subject seems to claim universal attention; and as there are particular situations and circumstances in which the ratio of advantage may be as three to two, and in some cases it may be double, its consideration ought to be proportionally incentive to individuals, to the obtaining the proposed end, where there is a probability of such circumstances existing.

These observations, united to the particular elucidation of the advantages derivable from a continued use of the Saccharometer, which is the subject-matter of the ensuing sheets, will, it is presumed,

be

be a sufficient inducement to the liberal,
the candid, and even the wary, to commence a satisfactory enquiry on the occafion, in the profecution of which there
is every thing to hope and nothing to
rifque.

STATICAL

STATICAL ESTIMATES

OF THE

MATERIALS FOR BREWING.

INTRODUCTION.

Containing the Defcription and Ufe of the Apparatus neceffary for conducting the Experiments.

I. *The* SACCHAROMETER, *its conftruction ana principles.*

THAT the bafis of this inftrument may not appear hypothetical, nor its application be deemed the refult of clofet fpeculation, to be trufted with caution by the man of bufinefs, a recital of the mode of its conftruction may be fatisfactory, to convince the timorous that in its adoption

he

he treads on fure ground, and to confirm the adventurous in the idea that the advantages promifed by the ufe of it, are founded on the fubftantial proofs of actual practice.

Having procured an inftrument to be made, according to particular inftructions, I adjufted the weight *(a)* at the bottom, *(fee the plate, fig.* 1.) fo as to occafion the inftrument to fink in the heavieft water I could procure, till the whole was immerfed except the upper part of the fcale, which was intended to be graduated downward from that part where the furface of the water reached *(b)*, and which was marked for that purpofe. I then put the inftrument into diftilled water, and it funk to the bottom; but the ftem being a tube, exactly fitted by the part to which the bottom weight was fcrewed, and which was fhut up, oh the firft immerfion of the inftrument, I drew this part a little way out of the tube *(c)*, by which the bulk of the inftrument was increafed without adding to its weight, and, by a little adjufting, it then funk no lower

in

in the distilled water, than it had sunk in the heavy water first made use of. The sliding part, of course, then became a *regulator*, by the drawing out or shutting up of which, the instrument might be made a counterpoise to any water fit for domestic use. This being noted, I pressed the regulator into the tube so far as that the instrument sunk to the point *(b)*, before indicated, in the river-water I employed for brewing, and thence becoming the equipoise or representative of that water, it was ready for my experiments.

It is here to be noted, that the water, in which the instrument was immersed, was always at fifty degrees of heat, by Fahrenheit's thermometer; and having adopted this temperature, as more stationary and more practicable than any other, I am altogether to be understood as referring to, or implying it, except where the contrary is expressly mentioned.

My next care was to provide a half barrel, as exact in its guage as I could procure, which having filled with river-

O   water,

water, I weighed it as accurately as the
weights I was neceffitated to employ
would admit of; and having deducted
the weight of the cafk, I found that of
the water to be 184½ pounds, or 369
pounds per barrel, of 36 gallons beer
meafure. I then filled the fame çafk
with my firft wort, previoufly cooled, and
found the net weight to be 204 pounds,
or 408 pounds per barrel, making an addition of 39 pounds to the weight of the
water; which experiments being repeated
in different worts, from each of which
fpecimens were faved, I proceeded to
apply the inftrument.

Having immerfed it in the firft wort, I
fixed an additional weight to the top *(d)*
of the fcale, which weight being adjufted
till the inftrument funk in the wort to the
extreme point *(b)* of the intended graduation, the additional weight immediately
became the reprefentative of the 39 pounds
additional denfity, acquired or extracted
by the water from the malt, in the fame
manner as the inftrument itfelf was, before,

fore, the reprefentative of the fimple element, whilft the combination of the inftrument, and its additional weight, reprefented the wort itfelf, confifting of water
and a quantity of extracted fermentable
matter equal to 39 pounds per barrel.

A fecond wort, weighed in the fame
manner, producing an addition of 21
pounds per barrel, I adjufted likewife a
weight for it, which weight was then the
reprefentative of that addition. Having
thus obtained the two weights 39 and 21,
I weighed them feparately, and reducing
the amount of each into grains, I found
they had a correfpondent relation to each
other; and, of courfe, that a weight equal
to the fum of them both, would be the
exact reprefentative of 60 pounds per barrel acquired denfity, at the fame time that
another of half that fum would reprefent
30. A confirmation of this was immediately obtained, by forming the weight 30,
according to this rule, and then mixing
equal parts of the two worts together, the
inftrument, on being immerfed therein

with

with that weight at the top, funk down to the point before indicated. In the fame manner 29 parts of this wort, and one of water, being mixed together, and a weight being formed equal to 29 parts of the 30, contained in the weight 30, the weight fo formed was fixed upon the inftrument when immerfed in the faid mixture, and it funk down as before, confirming thereby the truth of both, and eftablifhing a double fecurity for the accuracy of the experiments to be made with an inftrument conftructed upon thefe fimple principles.

In order to indicate the intermediate degrees, or parts of a pound, I immerfed the inftrument in the wort or mixture of 30 pounds per barrel, when the weight 29 only was applied, and preffing it down to the ufual point *(b)*, the finger was taken away, and the inftrument immediately emerged or rofe up, till the bulb was but juft covered with the liquor, the furface of which being then near the bottom of the fcale *(e)*, a mark was made at that point, and the fpace between that and the

upper

upper point *(b)*, being divided into ten equal parts, thòſe graduations were then ſo many one-tenth parts of a pound, be-cauſe the whole ſpace was equal thereto; for the weight 30 being applied, the in-ſtrument again ſunk to the upper point as before.

The penetrating eye of critical philoſo-phy will here readily perceive that this, though a broad and ſtrong foundation, every way adequate to the firm, rough ſtructure which the hand of buſineſs is to build upon it, is by far too rude a baſis for the finiſhed edifice, which philoſophi-cal inveſtigation might be inclined to erect thereon. Like ſtone, rough from the quar-ry, my unwieldy materials, though well enough adapted to the brewhouſe, were to undergo the operation of the chiſſel and ſquare before they could be admitted as the components of a building, whoſe bulk and proportion were to claim the attention of the public. The guage of my caſk could not be relied on as the accurate ad-meaſurement of its contents; nor, in the

ſituation

situation where the firft foundation of my
fyftem was laid, was it in my power to
procure any veffel whofe capacity was fo
truly afcertained, as to give with greater
precifion the contents of a barrel, upon
which, as a meafure univerfally applicable
to the bufinefs of the brewery, it was
thought proper to form my calculations.
As much, too, might be faid of my rude
half-hundred, quarter of a hundred, and
other weights, for whofe correctnefs I had
no better authority than that of the founder
who caft them. On thefe experiments, however, my firft inftrument was formed, and
I am happy to find that it varied very little
from that accuracy with which thofe now
offered to the public are made; the principles of which are formed on the niceft philofophical calculations and experiments, for
which I am indebted to the obliging of-
fices of a friend, whofe fituation enabled
him to procure fuch means of conducting
them as I could not have obtained; and
whofe judgment in applying them was,
I am confcious, fuperior to any capa-
bility

bility I could have called into action on the occasion. His manner of investigating the principles, and calculating the construction of the Saccharometer, as communicated by letter, contains so many judicious remarks, and displays so much ingenuity, that I am induced to subjoin the whole, by way of appendix, as a very probable gratification to the scientific reader, severely as it reflects on *the rudeness of my guage and weights*, to which, however, I have not been so much attached as to refuse the adoption of a more accurate system.

II. ASSAY JARS.

THESE need be nothing more than small tin vessels, *(see plate, fig. 2.)* of about eight inches long, and two or two and a half in diameter, with a small ear or handle at the top, somewhat like that of a common tin pot *(a)*. There may be six in number, in order to keep, till the brewing is finished, specimens of each wort, before and after boiling, if

curiosity

curiofity or any other motive fhould induce. Three of them, for the three un-
boiled worts, fhould have lids or covers
(b), the circle or rim of which muft fit
within the top of the jar, and not flip
over it on the outfide. The ufe of this
is to prevent the lofs of any of thofe aqueous particles, which will neceffarily evaporate at firft; but being arrefted and
condenfed by the lid, immediately trickle
down the fide, and by that means are again
conveyed into the wort from which they
arofe; whereas, if the lid flipped upon
the outfide of the jar, a great part of the
condenfed vapour would find its way between the infide of the rim of the lid, and
the outfide of the jar, and fo be loft.

III. JAR CASE.

A box 16 inches long, 12 inches broad,
and 7 deep, on the outfide, will be fufficient
for fix jars. It fhould be lined with milled
lead, in order to hold water; and through
the lid, which may be nailed faft down,
fhould

should be made six circular holes, about 2¼ inches diameter, in order to receive the six jars. *(See plate, fig. 3.)* These may be made three in a row, at equal distances from each other, and from the ends and sides of the box. A small lip or spout should be made from the upper part of the lead-lining, in order that the water may be the more readily poured out thereby; and that it may run over in that place only, in case of the box being accidentally filled too full. When intended for use, it is to be filled so full of cold water as just to admit the immersion of the six jars without running over.

IV. REFRIGERATOR.

THIS instrument may be made of tin, and being intended to contain no more than the quantity of an assay-jar full, its dimensions may be nine inches deep, and its breadth seven inches one way, and half an inch the other, forming a broad and flat or thin vessel, resembling a tin case sometimes made use of for the pre-

servation

fervation of deeds or other writings. (*See plate; fig.* 4.) The reafon of its being made thus thin, is, that when charged with hot wort, and plunged into cold water, the effect of the cold may be almoft inftantaneous, which is nearly the cafe; for the quantity of wort being lefs than a pint, and the furface brought into contact with the cold water (the intervention of the tin only excepted) containing very near 140 fquare inches, it may eafily be conceived how rapidly the heat muft be diffipated.

The upper part fhould have a lip (*a*) for the more conveniently pouring out the wort, and on the oppofite fide fhould be a focket, to which a handle (*b*) fhould be foldered. The ufe of the focket is to receive a ftick, of any convenient length (*c*), which is to fix in the focket by a pin, in the fame manner as a bayonet is fixed; by which means it may be faftened in, when the refrigerator is to be dipped into the copper, and taken out, as an incumbrance, when it is charged with wort.

It

It is to have two lids or covers, (*d* and *e*) the rims of which are to flip within the edge of the veſſel, as is recommended for thoſe of the aſſay-jars. One of the covers is to be perforated full of ſmall holes, in order to admit the wort, and at the ſame time to prevent the hops from entering; the other is to be whole, and is intended to ſupply the place of the firſt, the moment it is taken out of the copper.

The length of the ſtick, inſerted in the ſocket, is entirely to be determined by circumſtances, it being intended only as the means of holding the refrigerator in the wort, till it is filled, without endangering the hand from the ſteam.

It ſhould have a broad flat bottom (*f*), in order to enable it to ſtand upright, otherwiſe there would be a neceſſity of ſupporting it in that poſition.

STATICAL

STATICAL ESTIMATES

OF THE

MATERIALS FOR BREWING;

OR,

A TREATISE

ON THE

APPLICATION AND UTILITY

OF THE

SACCHAROMETER,

PART I.

Containing the Principles and Theory.

BEFORE I enter into a particular difcuffion of the utility of the Saccharometer, or attempt to direct its application, I fhall endeavour to explain and familiarize fuch few philofophical and technical terms, and fuch natural and
chemical

chemical operations, as unavoidably occur in the elucidation of a subject in
which both nature and art are busy agents,
Those to whom these subjects are already
familiar, will, I doubt not, have can-
dour enough to bear with patience the
recital of matters so well known to them,
when they reflect that my intention is
only to convey to those who know them
not, such information thereon as may facilitate and render effectual the application
of the instrument hereby offered to their
attention and practice.

SECTION I.

Of DENSITY *and* GRAVITY.

THE term *density* is applied to all
bodies, whether solid or fluid, in order
to convey an idea of their weight, in
relation to their bulk; so that any body
is said to be more or less dense than
another, when it contains more or less
weight in the same bulk. Thus a cubical
inch of standard silver being ten times

the

the weight of a cubical inch of rain water, is said to have ten times the density of that fluid. The discovery of this principle, as related to the doctrine of gravitation, and the laws of gravity, has been of infinite use to science in general, and to mechanics in particular. That commerce and the domestic arts have not been unbenefited hereby, may be evinced by its daily utility to the merchant and manufacturer, though that utility is unfortunately less beneficial than it might be, were the former more frequently to let commercial speculation embrace scientific, and the latter more generally to bid theory and practice walk hand in hand. There is not, perhaps, an article subject to the pursuit of commerce, whose value is not, mediately or immediately, determinable by its gravity; and it will readily be perceived, that the materials of the manufacturer, having once been the commodities of the merchant, have their value ascertainable by similar means. The goldsmith and lapidary can bear testimony to

the

the importance of this difcovery, in difcriminating the value of thofe rare articles which occupy their attention; and that objects of inferior worth are not made the fubjects of a like inveftigation, arifes from that inattention to things of daily occurrence, which feems to imply fo perfect a knowledge of their qualities, in every refpect, as to preclude the neceffity and propriety of all fcrutiny. Hence, to apply the fubject to our immediate purpofe, whilft the brewer is adjufting his balance to fcrutinize the demerits of a fweated guinea, his fervant, perhaps, in the execution of his unfcrutinized orders in the brewery, is wafting to the amount of feveral. That this arifes from a want of information in the doctrine which is our prefent fubject, will, I doubt not, be fufficiently evinced in the courfe of thefe pages. The farmer well knows that wheat of 70 pounds per bufhel will produce, in a certain proportion, more flour than that of 60, becaufe he can apply his fcales to the wheat before it is ground,

and

and to the flour when dressed. The brewer, in like manner, can tell that barley of 56 pounds per bushel will make better malt than that of 50, *cæteris paribus*; but when he comes to infuse it in water, he has no criterion to direct his judgment; his rule of proportion is drowned in the fluid, and he is necessitated to rest upon the vague determination of the palate, what I shall hereafter prove to be discriminable, to the greatest philosophical precision.

And this naturally leads me to the consideration of *gravity*, or that tendency which all bodies of greater density than the atmosphere have towards the centre of the earth; and as this tendency increases in proportion to the greater density of any body, the difference in this tendency, or, in other words, the different density of different bodies, compared with each other, is termed *specific gravity*; by the application of which term we are enabled to convey our ideas on the subject of the density of all bodies,

whether

whether folid or fluid, previoufly fixing upon fome body, of the leaft variable nature, as a ftandard of comparifon. Hence, making rain-water the ftandard, and calling it 1000, philofophers have communicated to us the denfity of every body which has been the fubject of their enquiries. Thus the denfity of pure gold, or rather its fpecific gravity, is faid to be 19,640, that of fine filver 11,091, that of lead 11,325, &c. &c. intimating, by the proportion which thefe numbers bear to 1000, that gold is near twenty times, and that filver and lead are more than eleven times heavier, or more denfe, than rain-water.

The means I have adopted of afcertaining, with accuracy, the value of the materials employed in brewing, through all thofe modifications in which the various parts of the procefs offer it to our notice, are fomewhat fimilar to thofe which have been ineffectually, becaufe inadequately, employed by others; the inftrument itfelf, though differing in principle, af-

Q   fuming

suming the general form of an *hydrometer*, by which the specific gravity of fluids is generally determined; but it is rather from the application than the form of the instrument, that the value of the information I am about to communicate is to be estimated.

The fluid which is the subject of our investigation, is, in the first instance, *water*, being the menstruum employed for the purpose of dissolving and extracting the saccharum and other valuable qualities of malt; which compound liquor, after extraction, receives the denomination of *raw wort*, and in that, its second state, demands a very attentive examination. The third predicament in which we find it claiming our attention, is in the state of *boiled wort*, being then more dense by decoction, and more heterogeneous by the addition of the essential qualities of hops, extracted during that operation. The fourth state of our fluid is that when, by a previous fermentation perfectly finished, it becomes a more uni-

form,

form, more homogeneous, and completely vinous liquor, generally termed *beer*, or
malt-liquor; which is the genus, of which
porter, amber, ale, and *beer* (the latter
particularly fo termed, whether *fmall* or
ftrong), are but fo many fpecies or dif-
tinctions, again fubdiftinguifhed by the
addition of the places moft celebrated for
their refpective production; as *London
porter, Burton ale, Dorchefter beer,* &c.
In the general practice of the brewery
the three former are all the fituations in
which there is a pofitive neceffity for the
application of the faccharometer; the
fourth being only of relative utility, having regard to the ftrength or degree of
fpirituofity generated by the action of fermentation, the difcovery of which has
long been wifhed for by thofe interefted
in the production of malt-liquor. And
this leads us to a fifth application of the
faccharometer upon our fluid in its pureft
and moft homogeneous ftate, viz. when,
by a final expofure to heat in the alem-
bic, it becomes a condenfed vapour, and

Q 2   is

is dignified by the appellation of *spirit*.
For this purpose an additional set of
weights would be requisite, when, by em-
bracing the business of the distiller, fresh
objects of pursuit, and fresh sources of
utility would present themselves, but not
unattended by additional difficulties in
directing its farther application.

That the use of this instrument bids
fairest to accomplish the desirable end of
ascertaining the strength of malt liquors,
will hereafter appear; and that this end
has not yet been accomplished is not to be
wondered at, since the very mode of producing them in perfection, common and
familiar as it appears in the eye of the
public, is in general but little understood *. The only attempt, or rather
profession, to ascertain their strength within
my knowledge, was that of a late celebrated philosopher, who, on publishing
an hydrometer for assaying spirituous liquors, roundly asserted in his treatise on

that

* See *Theoretic Hints on Brewing.*

that fubject, that it was " equally ufeful
in the difcovery of the ftrength of
domeftic liquors, fuch as *beer, ale,*
punch. &c. &c.* Thefe are his words, to
the beft of my recollection, as I quote by
memory. Unfortunately, however, for
the credit of his affertion, after I had
tried various forts of malt-liquor by it,
and found their fpecific gravities equally
various and difpruprotioned to their evident, though undefined ftrength, I applied to him for information on the method of ufing his inftrument, in order to
attain thefe ends, when he ingenuoufly
figned his recantation, in reply, by ac-
knowledging that " he knew of no inftru-
" ment which would difcover the ftrength
" of malt-liquors.' Being convinced, notwithftanding, that this difcovery muft be
involved in the doctrine of gravity, and
puzzled to find the denfity of fmall beer
equal or very little inferior to that of
ftrong, whilft the denfities of different
forts of beer exhibited a perfect chaos of
incongruity, it was not till after the cleareft

* See Martin's treatife on the *Hydrometer.*

eſt conviction, from much experience, of the very great utility derivable to the brewery from the application of an hydroſtatical inſtrument, that I formed the plan of the *Saccharometer*, and adapted the principles of it to every practicable part of the brewing proceſs, thence attaining the grand end of my enquiries, viz. *To trace the progreſs of vinous* SPIRIT, *from its firſt foundation or embryo, in the faccharine and other fermentable parts of the producing fluid, to its final iſſue, in a ſtate of perfection, from the ſtill.*

The theory of this proceſs is as follows: The menſtruum or water, employed by the brewer, becomes heavier or more denſe by the addition of ſuch parts of the materials as have been diſſolved or extracted by, and thence incorporated with it; the operation of *boiling*, and its ſubſequent *cooling*, ſtill adds to the denſity of it, by evaporation, (as will be hereafter explained) ſo that when it is ſubmitted to the action of fermentation, it is more denſe than at any other period.

In

In paffing through this operation of nature, a remarkable alteration takes place.
The fluid I am here fpeaking of, no fooner
begins to ferment than its denfity begins
to diminifh; and as the fermentation is
more or lefs perfect, the fermentable matter, whofe acceffion has been traced by the
increafe of denfity, becomes more or lefs
attenuated, and in lieu of every particle
thus attenuated, a fpirituous particle, of
lefs denfity than water, is produced; fo
that when the liquor is again in a ftate of
quietude, it is fo much fpecifically lighter
than it was before, as the action of fermentation has been capable of attenuating
the component parts of its acquired denfity; and, indeed, were it practicable to
attenuate the whole, the liquor would
become lighter or lefs denfe than water;
becaufe the quantity of fpirit produced
from and occupying the place of the fermentable matter, would diminifh the
denfity of the water in a degree bearing
fome proportion to that in which the latter had increafed it.

Hence

Hence it is evident that the strength of fermented liquors cannot be ascertained by the common doctrine of specific gravities, or a comparison of their density with that of the simple element employed in their production; but by a particular application of relative or *comparative gravity*, if it may be so termed; whence this general axiom may be established as a principle, viz. *That the attenuation of a given weight of fermentable matter, in any fluid, will produce a certain quantity of spirit; and that equal quantities of attenuated matter, in all fluids, whether of equal or different densities, will produce equal quantities of spirit, without any regard to the proportion which such attenuation may bear to the density of either.* The inference is obviously this: If the specific gravity of the fluid be noted immediately before fermentation, and again at any time after, when the operation has entirely ceased, the difference between the former and the latter will indicate the weight of fermentable matter attenuated; and, of course,

the

the quantity of fpirit produced. That this is approximating very nearly to the difcovery of what is termed *ftrength*, in fermented liquors, will not, I prefume, be difputed, but that it is not entirely competent to the end propofed, will be fhewn in its proper place.

From what has been faid on this fubject, it will readily be collected, that the great ufe of the faccharometer depends on noting the different denfity of any fluid in the different ftates wherein it may be found; or, in other words, the applying it, by the brewer, for the difcovery of the fpecific gravity of every wort, in order to determine what portion of the materials each has imbibed, thence to calculate an aggregate of the whole; and from a divifion of that aggregate into given portions, to effect an uniform regulation in the product; thereby reaping every advantage attainable from perfection of materials, or excellence of procefs, and avoiding every inconvenient effect refulting from contrary caufes.

The

The doctrine of the faccharometer, employed in this difcovery, is founded on the well-known theorem, that when a folid body is floating in any fluid, the part of the fluid difplaced by it is equal in bulk to fo much of the folid body as is immerfed in it, and equal in weight to the whole of that body. On this principle, the inftrument, being immerfed in water, fhould fink to a given point upon the fcale, (as indicated before) and there remain ftationary; but as the fpecific gravity of water is not every where the fame, the invention of the *regulator* has rendered the inftrument correctly applicable to every variety of water; for by drawing it outwards or preffing it inwards, till the inftrument finks to the required point in the water intended to be made ufe of, it then becomes the exact reprefentative of that water, and is fit for immediate application.

The inftrument being fo adjufted, the water is then the true ftandard of comparifon for our experiments; and if, on being

ing

ing immerfed in wort, it refufes to fink to
the fame point to which it defcended in
water, we are certain that the former is
more denfe than the latter, by the refiftance it makes to the defcending inftrument; and that if a weight added to the
top of the fcale caufes it to fink to the
point intended, the weight fo added muft
be the reprefentative of the fpecific gravity of the wort, or of the addition made
to the denfity of the water by the acceffion of fermentable matter, as has been
before intimated; for that part of the
fluid difplaced by the inftrument is ftill
the fame in bulk, but of greater denfity,
becaufe the part of the inftrument immerfed is of the fame magnitude, though
the inftrument itfelf is increafed in weight,
agreeably to the theorem juft quoted. To
afcertain this weight, fo as to give it an
immediate relative application to known
quantities of wort, is effential to the advantageous ufe of the inftrument, an illuftration of which has already been given
in treating of its conftruction.

In

In applying it to afcertain the ftrength of a fpirituous fluid, the effence or final ftate of perfection of all fermentable liquors, a new ftandard is to be fought for; and though the means of applying it are fimilar to thofe juft mentioned, the end or inference is diametrically oppofite; for in the former inftance increafed denfity is additional value, whereas in the prefent cafe, fpecific lightnefs, or rarity, is intrinfic worth; the one deriving its excellence from extraction, or the uniting to itfelf the effence of foluble bodies, the other from fublimation (if the term may be allowed) or the withdrawing itfelf pure, and, till condenfed, in an impalpable form, from the inveloping medium which was the bond of its union with the remaining parts of the fermented liquor which gave it exiftence.

As in the firft procefs the lighteft ftate of the fluid neceffarily becomes a ftandard, the fame rule is to be obferved in this; neverthelefs the ftandard for the latter is not fo eafily eftablifhed as that of the

former;

former; becaufe the governing fluid of
the firft is common to all the world,
whilft that of the laft is only obtainable
by the niceft chemical procefs, and when
obtained is vague and indefinite. The
fluid here alluded to is *alcohol*, a fpirit fo
highly rectified, and fo perfectly dephleg-
mated as to be totally *inflammable*; one
criterion of which is, that having gunpowder put into it, and being then fet on
fire, it will fo perfectly confume itfelf as
at laft to fire the gunpowder, which it
could not do were the leaft particle of
aqueous moifture to remain in it. But as
this ftate of total inflammability may have
various degrees of perfection, and as two
quantities of alcohol may be different in purity, and yet may be both capable of firing
gunpowder, or of ftanding the teft of other
criterions, this ftandard muft be, in fome
degree, indefinite, till a more perfect mode
of afcertaining its purity fhall be difcovered. In general, however, it means the
pureft product of the moft perfect diftillation, or the lighteft palpable fluid which

can

ean be produced. Hence alcohol is made the ftandard of purity on one hand, water the boundary of impurity on the other, and the medium or commixture of equal parts of both is termed *proof fpirit*. This commixture, therefore, as a ftate in which all fpirits are moft applicable to domeftic purpofes, is ever made the meafure by which their value is eftimated; fo that if any fpirituous liquor be lighter or ftronger than this medium, it is termed *above proof*; if weaker, *below proof*; and their relative eftimates are determined by the abounding portion of alcohol in the one, and by its deficiency, or the abounding portion of water in the other. Thus fpirits are faid to be *one to three, four,* or *five*, or fo many *per cent.* over proof; or, on the contrary, under proof in a like definite proportion; meaning, by the former, that it would require one gallon of water to be added to fo many gallons of the fpirit fo eftimated, or fo many gallons of water to one hundred of fpirit, to bring it to the ftandard of *proof fpirit*. By the latter,

latter, or the same modes of expression applied to under proof, it is meant that the water is abundant in those several proportions, and that it would, of course, require such quantities of alcohol to be added, in order to raise it to the point of proof spirit above-mentioned; in both cases making due allowance for the concentration * of the commixture.

In assaying these fluids, being of less specific gravity than water, it would be necessary that the saccharometer should be reduced in weight, (which is effected by changing the weight at the bottom) so as to be the exact counterpoise of alcohol, when

* By *concentration* is meant that principle, in the commixture of two fluids of such different gravities, as water and alcohol, by which the particles of the one commix or fit so closely with those of the other, as to occupy a less space when united than they did separate. For instance, 50 gallons of water and 50 gallons of alcohol, when mixed together, do so far blend, incorporate, or *concentrate*, that the whole commixture will fall considerably short of 100 gallons; and of course the number of gallons of water or spirit, to be added to bring the fluid to proof spirit, will vary in that proportion.

when immerfed therein, as it was that of water before the alteration. In this cafe it would be ready, with the addition of requifite weights for the top, as before mentioned, to inveftigate and afcertain, with the greateft accuracy, every degree of impurity exifting in any fpirituous fluid, by the fimple comparifon of its fpecific gravity with that of water. For if the inftrument itfelf, immerfed to the required point, be then the reprefentative of alcohol, and the additional weight at the top, which finks it to the fame point in water, be termed 100, and that weight be divided into 100 parts, it necefarily follows that 50, or the one half of that weight, will be the reprefentative of proof fpirit; and that one, or a fingle divifion, will indicate to the one hundredth, whilft the ten intermediate graduations on the fcale, will fhew to fo fmall a degree as the one-thoufandth part, the quantity of water contained in the fluid.

To attain, however, that accuracy of which an inftrument thus conftructed is capable, it would be necefary to attend

tend to a particular which feems hitherto
to have efcaped the notice of thofe who
have offered hydrometers to the public;
and this is to afcertain the extreme point
of comparifon, or the fpecific gravity of
the water intended to form that point,
with the greateft poffible precifion. In
an *unmixed fpirit*, the intermediate weights
fhould be fubdivifions of that which
would immerfe the inftrument in diftilled water; but thefe will not anfwer the
intention if the fpirit has been mixed with
common water; for, in that cafe, the extreme point of comparifon, oppofed to
alcohol, being changed, the weights
would be no longer proportional parts of
that ftandard, and every experiment made
therewith muft be inaccurate.

To conduct thefe experiments with the
required precifion, we are to take particular care that the heat of the fluid be always the fame, at the time of applying
the inftrument, or that fuch allowances
be made, as experience fhall authorize to
be equivalent to thofe effects which heat

S   is

is known to produce in all bodies, ever expanding them in proportion to its own force and their ſuſceptibility of it ; ſo that the denſity of the ſame body is not the ſame in a warm as it is in a cold ſituation, but varies accordingly as the heat varies to which it is expoſed ; and without including the conſideration of theſe effects in the doctrine of denſity, all our experiments relative thereto, and all our inferences drawn therefrom, would be erroneous and fallacious, as will be more fully indicated in the following ſection.

SECTION II.

Of EXPANSION *and* CONTRACTION.

It is a well known axiom that all bodies *expand* with heat, and *contract* with cold; or that a body of a certain bulk, at a certain degree of heat, will be increaſed in magnitude in a greater heat, and be diminiſhed in a leſs. In ſolid bodies this principle generally receives the denomination,

tion of *expansion*, in the former instance, and of *contraction* in the latter; but in fluids these terms are, with great propriety, changed into *rarefaction* and *condensation*; because in the first case the fluid is rendered more *rare*, or of less specific gravity, and in the last it becomes more *dense*, or of greater gravity, than it was in the state which is made the point of comparison. But as these terms relate rather to the quality or confistence of the fluid than to the volume of it, I shall adopt the former on the present occafion, as more applicable to our purpose.

Dr. Halley, it is said, found that boiling water expanded one twenty-sixth part of its former bulk, though in a moderate heat its expansion was imperceptible; and by the same authority we are told that spirit of wine expands one twelfth part of its bulk, at that degree of heat at which it boils; the obvious inference is, that the lighter the fluid the greater the expansion at the same degree of heat; and in the two fluids here quoted the difference is

very

very great, since it is to be considered that spirit of wine boils at 176, by Fahrenheit's thermometer, and water at 212.

For the purpose of establishing my system on a firm basis, not of contending with so great an authority, nor of wandering in fields of philosophy unwarranted by an attention to my own pursuits, I was necessitated to enter upon an examination of the expansion of the same simple fluid which forms the subject of one of the doctor's experiments, and which I found to be so correspondent, that at 200 degrees it had expanded 3.5 per cent. or near one twenty-eighth part; but the ebullition then became too violent to make an accurate observation at any higher degree. It is with the utmost deference, also, that from observations on my own experiments I am led to enquire, by what means the expansion of a fluid could be accurately ascertained in a state of ebullition, when every part is in evident and violent motion, as well as in a state of copious evaporation? and how the above doctrine

came

came to be eftablifhed, "that the lighteft "fluids are fufceptible of the greateft ex- "panfion?" My own experiments unfortunately tend to confirm me in a contrary opinion; but as I am folicitous that this opinion fhould not be deemed to owe its exiftence to hypothefis, I will attempt to defcribe the manner of conducting thofe experiments on which it is founded.

Having procured a glafs tube of one inch diameter *(a)*, and 13 inches long, *(fee plate, fig. 5.)* I caufed it to be inferted, by means of an external focket, in the centre of the convex top of a cylindrical tin veffel *(b)*, capable of containing fomewhat lefs than ten times the quantity which was contained in a depth of ten inches of the tube. The reafon of its containing *fomewhat lefs* than ten times the quantity of ten inches in the tube, was, that being charged with that quantity of water, it might rife up a little way into the tube itfelf; fo that fixing a fcale of ten inches, fubdivided into tenths, to the tube, and commencing the graduation at the

furface

surface of the water, the length of the whole scale then became the exact measure of the one-tenth part of the water in the vessel, whilst every inch indicated the one-hundredth, and every tenth the one-thousandth part of it; a degree of accuracy beyond which I thought it unnecessary to proceed. In another part of the cover I inserted and supported a thermometer *(c)*, the bulb of which went sufficiently deep into the vessel, to indicate the heat of the fluid it contained; and the scale was fixed parallel to the tube and scale of the vessel, that observations might conveniently be made on them both at the same instant. The machine being thus prepared, it became, in some measure, a thermometer within a thermometer; for as the heat of the fire, on which it was placed, acted upon the fluid in which the bulb of the thermometer was immersed, the expansion of the fluid in the one, and of the mercury in the other, took place at the same time; and, of course, the former ascended in the tube of the machine,

chine, in proportion as the latter rofe in that of the thermometer. By this means I have been able to afcertain the expanfion of water, and that of worts of every probable denfity, and at every practicable degree of heat; whence I find, in direct oppofition to the above-quoted authority, that the expanfion of worts (whatever may be the effect of lefs heterogeneous fluids) increafes as they increafe in denfity, and that very nearly in the ratio of their fpecific gravities; for, in a prepared wort, (ftronger perhaps than any ever extracted from malt only) whofe fpecific gravity, compared with water, was nearly as 7 to 6, the expanfion was as 3.9 to 3.5 per cent. and my experiments made on feveral worts of intermediate denfities were entirely correfpondent, as will appear from the *Table of Expanfion* given with the faccharometer.

In the application of this doctrine to worts, which from the commencement to the conclufion of the brewing procefs, and confequently in every point of obfervation,

tion, are in a state of heat various but always superior to that which has necessarily been established as a standard for the instrument, we are immediately led to enquire, what will be the variation in the volume of a wort of any given gravity and quantity, at different degrees of heat, when contracted by that degree of comparative cold which I call the standard temperature?

It is also necessary for us to determine, under the same variation of circumstances, what is the sum of the acquired density of, or the quantity of fermentable matter incorporated with, every extract; but the instrument with its weights, being only capable of indicating the gravity of a fluid at a certain fixed degree of heat, it follows of course that an experiment made with it at any other degree, does only exhibit the gravity of that fluid at that particular degree of heat, and not what it would be at the temperature of the standard. Whence the *table of heat*, attending the instrument, is indispensably necessary,

to

to reduce every probable gravity at every practicable degree of heat, to the defired ftandard, in order to fhew the true fpecific gravity of every extract; and the *table of expanfion* becomes equally neceffary, to point out, in the fame gravities and degrees of heat, the exact volume or *quantity* of the fluid when contracted to the fame ftandard; by the affiftance of which we are enabled to afcertain the fum or aggregate of the acquired denfity, or the amount of the fermentable matter extracted. To exemplify this, I will fuppofe the inftrument fhewed the fpecific gravity of a fluid to be 50, at 100 degrees of heat, and that the fame fluid, at 50 degrees, was found by the fame inftrument to be 53, which is really the cafe, a calculation founded on the former experiment, without regard to the latter, would be erroneous in a ratio of 6 per cent. Again, if a proper attention has been paid to the above circumftance, and we fuppofe 53 to be the true fpecific gravity of a certain portion of wort, the whole quantity of

T

which

which is 100 times that portion, guaged when at 150 degrees, which is a probable heat; without reference to the *table of expansion*, we should immediately multiply 53 by 100, calling 5300 the aggregate density, or amount of the fermentable matter of the whole wort, thereby causing an error of near two per cent. for, by the table just mentioned, it appears that 100 of a fluid of this density, at 150 degrees of heat, are, in fact, not much more than 98 at 50 degrees; whence the aggregate error, in this case, would be as 5194 is to 5300, or the valuation of the wort would be false to the amount of 106 parts in 5300. And, as the examples I am now giving allude to the experiments on the newly-drawn extracts in the under back, upon the correctness of which the certain regulation of the *length* depends, it behoves us to be particularly careful not to draw inferences from false premises, and thence build an important structure upon an unsound foundation.

To

To a philofophical reader it will readily occur, that expanfion is not the only principle to be confidered in the conduct-ing thefe experiments; for though the introduction of heat into a folid body, tends only to a feparation of its parts, fo as to caufe the expanfion of the whole; and though the re-union of thofe parts, and the confequent contraction of the whole, to its former ftate and bulk, is the immediate effect of the withdrawing of the heat fo introduced; yet a fluid having un-dergone the fame procefs, neither refumes its original volume nor denfity, on a return to its original temperature, but the former is diminifhed, and the latter increafed; an effect ever produced by that diminution of quantity to which every fluid has a tendency, when expofed to a degree of heat fuperior to that of itfelf in a tempe-rate ftate of the air; for the expanfion of a fluid, or a partial feparation of its com-ponent parts by heat, is ever attended by a total efcape of fuch of them as are fuffi-ciently volatile to be carried off by their mutual repulfion of each other, thereby

caufing

causing that diminution of quantity and additional density just alluded to; a farther illustration of which will be the business of the subsequent section.

SECTION III.

Of EVAPORATION,

THE general definition of evaporation, is that effect of heat whereby the lighter particles of a fluid, to which heat is applied, are separated from the rest, and fly off into the air, in the form of vapour, by which means the remainder becomes of a more dense consistency; or, if the separation be carried to the last extremity, some fluids will assume a solid form, and others will fly off entirely. The theory of this principle may be thus explained: In proportion as the heat insinuates itself into the body of the fluid, the particles of which it consists have a tendency to separate from each other; and when the heat becomes sufficiently strong,

ſtrong, this ſeparation actually takes place; at which period, the particles thus ſeparated, becoming mutually repellent, riſe from the ſurface of the fluid in a body, at equal diſtances from each other; and being hence ſpecifically lighter than the ſame bulk of airy particles, riſe up into the atmoſphere like a cloud, till they reach that part which is of the ſame degree of rarity with themſelves, unleſs arreſted and condenſed in their paſſage, by ſome intervening ſolid, which cauſes their re-union and return to that ſtate, collectively, in which ſeparately their avolation began. Thoſe which do actually riſe into the air, as juſt mentioned, remain ſuſpended or ſtationary no longer than their acquired heat, and conſequent rarefaction continues; but as that becomes leſs, their repellent force decreaſes; the immediate conſequence of which is, their deſcent in that progreſſion which their re-union and condenſation, or returning denſity, render unavoidable; ſtill

ſinking

finking as they become more denfe, till of neceffity they return to the earth.

On all fluids produced by chemical proceffes, the action and effect of evaporation are the fame, i. e. the avolation or efcape of the lighter particles, whereby that part of the fluid which remains is infpiffated, or rendered of a more denfe confiftence than the whole was before the commencement of this action; but though the pofitive effect is the fame, its relative confequence differs according to the nature of the fluid which is its fub-ject; and as all chemical fluids may be claffed under the two general heads of *extracts* and *effences,* this difference of relative effect may be explained, by ob-ferving that evaporation tends to melio-rate or enrich the former, and to injure or impoverifh the latter. By the term *extracts* I would be underftood to mean all artificial fluids impregnated with the diffoluble parts of folid bodies, either by decoction or fimple infufion; and all na-tural fluids, fuch as vegetable juices, ob-

tainable

tainable by fpontaneous extraction or ex-
preffion. By *effences* I would convey
an idea of fluids, which have been the
fubject of fermentation, whereby their heterogeneous particles are affimilated, and
in fome meafure rendered homogeneous ;
or of diftillation, whereby the greateft degree of purity is effected which art can
produce.

On the firft mentioned fpecies of fluid,
evaporation having only the power of
feparating the aqueous parts, its certain
effect is, a nearer approach, or more intimate union of the extracted parts of
the diffolved body, on which its value depends, whence it gains in gravity what
it lofes in bulk ; for the fum of its valuable particles remains the fame, though
the volume of the fluid is diminifhed.
On the other hand, all vinous fluids, the
refult of fermentation, and all diftilled
liquors, receive irreparable injury from
evaporation ; becaufe the value of every
fermented and diftilled fluid, confifting in
its moft volatile parts, an expofure to this
action,

action, in causing their separation, deprives the fluid of the principle which constitutes its worth, and leaves it at length a mere caput mortuum. Common observation will confirm these different effects; for daily experience shews us, that by long exposure to the air only, a saccharine mixture will become a syrup, sea water evaporate to salt, wine and beer lose their spirituosity and become vinegar, and distilled liquors retain only the simple element which formed their basis.

So far as the doctrine of evaporation is evinced by the visible effect of *steam*, arising from every heated fluid, it will be comprehended by all ranks and capacities; but to trace its efficient causes *ab origine*, to measure its relative influences, and to deduce its final consequences, requires a degree of philosophical reflection which few people, engaged in commercial pursuits, find either the leisure or inclination to bestow. In the brewery, though this active principle is ever before the artist's eyes, he is generally as little acquainted with

with its effects as if none exifted; whence arife many difagreeable and difadvantageous errors, which, it is hoped, an attention to thefe pages will effectually remove.

In order to apply the faccharometer for this end, we are previoufly to confider the different ftates and local fituations in which the fluid to be affayed is necef-farily found; the relative predicament in which the portion intended for the immediate fubject of experiment ftands; and the inference to be drawn from a comparative view of the whole.

The firft of thefe confiderations includes *extraction,* or the withdrawing tho liquor from the impregnating materials, and the confequent fituation of the extract in the under-back. Secondly, *decoction,* or the operation of boiling that extract in the copper. And laftly, *refrigeration,* or the act of expofing a very large furface of the boiled wort in the cooler, preparatory to its being fermented.

U   With

With respect to extraction, or more properly the situation of the wort immediately subsequent to that part of the process, it were superfluous to note the effect of evaporation during its continuance in that state; because, what we want to ascertain there, is the acquired density of the whole, and not the specific gravity of a part, no farther than as that specific gravity is instrumental in ascertaining the aggregate density.

During the action of boiling, the effect of evaporation is not less critical than important; because, the due division of the aggregate density into the intended equal portions, or the certain regulation of the length, depends very much thereon. For the quantity evaporated in the cooler may, in a great measure, be ascertained, since it generally bears a certain proportion to the whole wort turned out of the copper, including some consideration for the extent of the surface exposed; but in the great uncertainty which attends the vapour arising out of a fluid in a state of violent ebullition,

ebullition, we have no other means of determining the quantum evaporated, at any
period of the operation, than by learning
the then specific gravity of the given equal
portion, which divided in the aggregate
densobserve, will give the number of those
portions remaining at that period, and,
of course, ascertain the amount of the evaporation; for instance, if there were sixteen of these portions in the extract, and
we call the specific gravity three, the aggregate density will be forty-eight; and if
at any period of the action of boiling we
find by experiment, that the specific gravity be four, by dividing that in forty-eight
we know that the number of portions remaining is twelve, and consequently that
four are evaporated. Were there no intervening obstacle to the immediate application of this doctrine, the rule would be
general, and the event certain; but as
such occurrences do necessarily and at all
times exist, in practice, their consideration
is indispensable, before any accurate con-

U 2 clusions

clufions can be drawn, or any correct eftimate made, as will appear hereafter.

The two preceding circumftances being only of relative ufe, as conducive to
the perfect regulation of the final unfermented ftate of the wort, the confideration
of them is only prefented as an object to
be kept in view, in order with greater certainty to direct us to that final average
gravity, which is the ultimate eventual
confequence of all the evaporations to
which the wort has been expofed, and
particularly the immediate effect of that
which refults from refrigeration, or the
act of cooling. As the quantum or amount
of this laft evaporation may be with fufficient accuracy afcertained; as the event
is pofitive, and admits of no real or ad-
miffible correction; and as the effect of
decoction or boiling has an immediate
governing influence on it; we may thence
collect, that it is of the laft importance
to the intended regulation of the *length*, or
final average gravity required, to bring
the wort into the cooler in fuch a ftate as
will

will produce that gravity, after the laſt evaporation has taken place.

To exemplify this, by enlarging on the caſe above quoted, I will ſuppoſe that from the ſixteen given portions of the extract, whoſe ſpecific gravity is three, and whoſe aggregate denſity is forty-eight, it were required to produce a ſtandard wort, whoſe ſpecific gravity, in a fermentable ſtate, ſhall be ſix, it immediately occurs (without including the intervening obſtacles before alluded to) that the whole evaporation muſt amount to one half of the wort; becauſe ſix divided in forty-eight produces eight, which is the number of portions remaining after the aqueous particles ſhall have been ſo far evaporated as to leave the ſpecific gravity of the wort at ſix. Now if we eſtimate the poſitive and unavoidable evaporation which takes place during the paſſage of the wort from the copper to the cooler, including its continuance therein, at a one-ninth part of the whole, we can directly calculate the quantum of wort which

which ought to be in the copper, at the time of its being turned out, by saying, as eight (the intended volume of cold wort) is to nine, (the quantum of hot) so is any other intended quantity of cold wort, to its proportionate quantity of hot. This, in the present case, is nine parts of the original sixteen, because the quantum intended to be finally remaining is eight. Then, in order to calculate the specific gravity of the wort, when evaporated to those nine parts or portions, we are to divide forty-eight, the aggregate density, by nine, the required quantum of hot wort, and the quotient is 5.33, which denotes the specific gravity the wort ought to have when ready to be turned out of the copper, in order to produce the required specific gravity, or strength of the wort in the cooler, in a fermentable state.

This elucidation naturally includes an attention to a particular before mentioned, i. e. the relative predicament in which the specimen stands, which is taken out for the purpose of experiment, and which may be a false representation of the wort

it

it was taken from, owing to the different effects of evaporation in different situations of the evaporating fluid, as will be more particularly shewn in its place. In all cases, the wort is to be guaged and the specimen taken at the same time, except in boiling wort, where the experiment is made merely for the purpose of ascertaining the quantity at that instant, as above explained; and in every state of the wort, the business is to be done at the very last period of its continuance in that particular state which is the subject of investigation. In the under-back, it has no other use than to prevent any addition (by farther draining from the mash-tun) from being made to the quantity of the wort after the guage and specimen are taken; for the business required here being only to ascertain the sum of the acquired density, and evaporation having no effect upon that, it is of no immediate consequence, whether the same be continued in a rarefied, or be reduced into a condensed state, or contracted volume, so long

as

as the assay-jar, by being closed at the top, to prevent evaporation, preserves a perfect specimen of what the wort in the under-back would have been, at a similar degree of heat, had no evaporation taken place.

The experiment on the wort in the copper requires some little dexterity, to conduct it with efficacy and dispatch. The quantity of wort taken out, as a specimen, by the refrigerator, and plunged into cold water, to reduce it to an assayable heat, should, with all possible expedition, be submitted to the examination of the instrument; for a repetition of this being necessary, at different periods of the boiling, were the experiments to take up much time, the copious evaporation which takes place during that action, might risque an increase of the specific gravity beyond the intended degree, and so defeat the very purpose of the enquiry.

A similar attention is necessary to the time of taking the specimen for experiment on the wort in the coolers, (the particulars of which will be given in the

practical

practical directions) left by the evaporation of the affay-jar, if the fpecimen be taken hot, being inferior to that of the cooler, the wort in the former fhould be a falfe reprefentation of that in the latter; inafmuch as it would, in that cafe, be fpecifically lighter, and occafion an error difadvantageous to the brewer, who, on this occafion, has nothing to aim at but the production of his ftandard fpecific gravity, as a foundation for the ftandard ftrength of his liquor; which if he exceed, it is to his pofitive lofs; and of which, if he fall fhort, it is to his immediate difcredit, and to his eventual difadvantage.

Having now, I prefume, fufficiently explained the three grand principles whofe agency is moft powerful in the bufinefs which is the fubject of our enquiries, I proceed to inveftigate the qualities of the materials which are to form the bafis of our experiments.

SECTION

SECTION IV.

Of the FERMENTABLE MATTER *extractible from* MALT.

THE value of malt confifting in its diffoluble parts, and thefe being obtainable in different proportions, according to the quality of the barley employed, or the fkill of the maltfter in conducting the procefs of its vegetation, it is matter of furprife that fome certain means have not before been invented to regulate what the brewers term the *length* (i. e. the quantity of beer to be made from a given quantity of malt), rather by the *quality* than by the *quantity* of the malt made ufe of. When the brewer fays he draws one and a half, two, two and a half, or three barrels from a quarter of malt, it means no more than that he employs fo much malt to make fo much beer, without conveying any determinate idea of the quality of either. He may, indeed, premife that his malt is of a good, bad, or indifferent
rent

rent quality, for the fake of diftinction, and yet we are left to make a very vague guefs at the refult of its application; for the terms *good* and *bad* are totally indefinite, unlefs applied in reference to a ftandard eftablifhed on the broad bafis of mathematical certainty. In the prefent cafe, an inftrument which will afcertain the quantity of the diffoluble parts, or of the fermentable matter extracted from malt of every kind, will not only difcriminate its value, but point out the value of the liquor produced from it, in explicit and communicable terms. This is what the brewer has long wanted; for though he could tell that ftronger beer might be made from better malt, or from a greater quantity of the fame malt, yet he has ever been at a lofs to determine in what proportion it would be better, were fuch fuperiority or addition to take place. The inftruments hitherto publifhed, with the view of affifting him herein, have been totally incompetent to the purpofe. Many reafons might be adduced in fup-

port

port of this affertion, without derogating
from the ingenuity of the inventors or
publifhers; but one will fuffice :—They
were the attempts of men, who, not pof-
feffing the means of information adequate
to the end propofed, could have no applicable foundation whereon to build a
fyftem of that certain and complete utility
which the fubject requires, and of which
it is capable.

The inftrument now offered to the
public, by fhewing how many pounds
avoirdupois of fermentable matter are
contained in every barrel * of wort extracted from the malt, leads immediately to the difcovery of what portion of
the latter has been imbibed by, or incorporated with the extracted menftruum,
and of courfe, what has been the product
or intrinfic value of every quarter of
malt employed; pointing out, at the
fame time, how much of that product
is contained in a barrel of wort in a fer-

X 2   mentable

* Thirty-fix gallons, beer meafure, as before
explained.

mentable ftate, whether entire or a commixture of feveral; thence eftablifhing a
mathematical definition, which conveys
pofitive ideas on the fubject, and cannot
be mifunderftood.

By the long-continued ufe of this inftrument, in my own practice, as well
as from its occafional application elfewhere, I am authorifed to pronounce it
the moft ufeful, becaufe the moft advantageous inftrument the brewer can
adopt. The difcoveries it has laid open
to my view, have been of fo interefting
a nature, that I have often been ftruck
with aftonifhment to find that common
obfervation and attention fhould be fo inadequate to the purpofe of fecuring or
obtaining of very important advantages
derivable from a very common profeffion,
which has been fo long involved in darknefs and error, as to create a vulgar opinion that it neither requires nor admits
of fcience nor fyftem.

In the courfe of my experiments I have
found, that by means of the faccharometer,

ter, I am enabled to eſtimate the intrinſic worth of every kind of malt, to
the very great preciſion of the one-thou-
ſandth part of the fermentable matter extracted from every quarter employed.
And by eſtimates made in this manner,
I have diſcovered a great variety in malts,
which, but for theſe diſcoveries, would
ſcarcely have been deemed of different
value. From ſuch as have fallen under
my obſervation in practice, during the
three years preceding the firſt publication
of this treatiſe, I have ſelected the following, the reſpective value of which
will be known by the ſum of the fermentable matter ſeverally extracted from
them.

MALT *from the barley of* 1781.

Nº	Colour.	Character.	Growth of barley.	Average prod. of ferm. matter
1	pale	well made	North Lincolnſh.	82 pounds
2	ditto	indifferent	ditto — —	75 ditto
3	ditto	well made	Norfolk —	72 ditto
4	ditto	ditto —	Yorkſh. woulds	82 ditto
5	brown	ditto —	ditto — —	78 ditto
6	ditto	ditto —	Ware, in Herts.	56 ditto

MALT

MALT *from the barley of* 1782.

Nº	Colour.	Character.	Growth of barley	Average prod.
1	pale	well made	Yorkſh. woulds	62 pounds
2	ditto	ditto —	Bremen — —	58 ditto
3	ditto	ditto, —	Norfolk — —	67 ditto
4	ditto	indifferent	ditto —. —	56 ditto
5	brown	well made	Ware, in Herts.	54 ditto

MALT *from the barley of* 1783.

Nº	Colour.	Character.	Growth of barley.	Average prod.
1	pale	well made	North Lincolnſh.	74 pounds
2	ditto	ditto —	Berwick on Tweed	63 ditto
3	ditto	indifferent	Yorkſh. woulds	65 ditto
4	ditto	well made	ditto — —	75 ditto
5	brown	ditto —	ditto — —.	72 ditto

The average products above-quoted are all deduced from the different produce of different brewings, made from the ſame parcel of malt, which ſometimes varied a few pounds from the reſpective averages here ſtated; and this variation might ariſe from an eſſential difference in the malt itſelf, owing to the different degrees of perfection to which the vegetative proceſs of different floors might have arrived, though conſiſting of the ſame kind of barley;

ley; or it might result from the difference
in grinding the same malt rounder at one
time than at another; for the intention of
malting being the production of that faccharum, and other diffoluble parts * which
conftitute the value of malt, it follows, of
courfe, that in proportion as that procefs
approaches to perfection, the increafe of
thofe valuable parts will be effected; and
as the crufhing of every kernel in pieces
is indifpenfable to the fetting at liberty its
fermentable matter, it is obvious that if
the operation of grinding be fo carelefsly
performed, that a certain number pafs
•through the ftones unbroken, the product
muft be lefs in the proportion which thefe
bear to the whole volume. Hence a continued attention is neceffary to thefe preliminary particulars, as a foundation for
thofe advantages which are to refult from
pofterior confiderations.

The different products of the different
fpecimens above-ftated convey important
information to the brewer, and fuggeft a
vaft field of beneficial enquiry. By thofe

we

* *See Theoretic Hints on Brewing*

we fee that good pale malt, from ftout barley, will produce, in the ordinary mode of practice, 82 pounds of fermentable matter; and this produce the barley of moft of the inland counties is capable, and that of fome will exceed it. We alfo fee, in the fourth and fifth articles of the year 1781, that brown (not *blown)* malt produces 78 pounds per quarter, made from the fame barley, and by the fame procefs of vegetation, which in pale produces 82; and that the Hertfordfhire barley, in the fixth article, generally fuperior to that alluded to, made into brown malt, by the Ware practice, produces only 56. By the former practice, there is a deficiency in the produce of brown malt, of about 5 per cent. by the latter the lofs is more than 30; a difference fo very great, that were it not mathematically demonftrable, credibility would be ftaggered at an affertion which feems fo feverely to reflect on the judgment of many people, whofe predilection for Ware malts has been of long ftanding, particularly in London, where

Y   they

they are most fought after, and bear the best price. It is, indeed, with the utmost respect, that I submit to the confideration of the gentlemen who stand in this predicament, the difference here announced between brown malts dried in the common method, and those which are *blown* by the precipitate mode practifed at Ware and its environs.

Independent of the demonstration of this error by the faccharometer, I need only appeal to the understanding of any perfon, whether he be converfant or not in the nature of malt, to bear testimony of its existence, however indefinite in degree it may be found, in the want of the demonstrative means here alluded to. For were fuch a common obferver to be informed, that every kernel of blown malt is of a magnitude exceeding the bulk of the barley from which it was made, in a ratio of four to three, or thereabouts, and that this excefs of magnitude is occafioned only by a rarefaction of the air within, arifing from a fudden application of violent
lent

lent heat to the green malt, which puffs up the outer fkin like a bladder filled with air, in which ftate it is fixed by the continuance of the heat, he will immediately conclude, that the cavity found in every kernel, though it may very well ferve to buoy up its fellow, and fill the buſhel, will produce no fermentable matter in the maſh-tun ;—*ex nihilo nil fit.*

It may be farther obferved, on the defects of brown malts in general, compared with pale made from the fame fpecies of barley, that the procefs of brewing porter, and other beers, in which a portion of brown malt is necefſarily introduced, is more productive of fermentable matter than that which common ufage has adopted where pale malts only are employed; the rational inference of this is, that the real deficiency of the former is greater than it appears to be in the experiments adduced; becaufe the products therein ftated are thofe of the different procefſes juft alluded to, and not comparative views of the products refulting from

Y 2   the

the fame procefs ; a circumftance which, in the practical and feparate ufe of brown and pale malts, very rarely occurs.

From the above view of the malts pro- duced from the barley of 1781, which was in a ftate of general perfection, much more ufeful information may be collected. The two firft articles are fpecimens of the produce of the fame kind of barley, under the management of two different malt- fters. In the former there is a fuperiority over the latter of nine per cent. a confi- derable difference, to an amount which, in moft commercial concerns, is deemed a fair profit ; and yet thefe two parcels of malt would have paffed, among common confumers, with this fimple obfervation that *this fample is freer than that*; the difference in fale, would not, perhaps, have exceeded a fhilling per quarter ; and the brewer would have thrown them in- difcriminately into the mafh- tun, drawing his ufual length from each, to the pofitive lofs of 9 per cent. either in the quality of his liquor from the latter parcel, or in the

obtainable

obtainable profits of his trade from the former; which ever might happen to tally with the general quality of the malt he ufed.

The third article leads us to the detection of an error generally prevalent in the northern parts of the kingdom, which is the preference given there to Norfolk barley. Yet this preference has a very rational foundation, fo far as it is found to be more vegetative, or to *malt more freely* than the native barley of thofe parts. Neverthelefs, this is too often to be attributed more to the ignorance of the maltfter, than to the quality juft mentioned. If the fpecimen here quoted (made from a fair parcel of Norfolk barley, under the infpection of a friend, whofe knowledge of the malting bufinefs is very extenfive) be compared with that made from the Lincolnfhire barley in the firft article, we fhall find a difference in favour of the latter of 12½ per cent. and furely no perfon, after fuch a demonftration, would be weak enough to give a fuperior price

for

for a commodity deficient in value to so
confiderable an amount.

The barley of the year 1782, prefents
us with a melancholy fpectacle of the
effects of that ungenial feafon. The firft
article exhibits the produce of the fame
maltfter, occupied upon barley from the
fame place which is quoted in the fourth
article of the preceding year, and " what
" a falling off is there!" —an advance of
100 per cent. in price, with a reduction in
quality of near 24 per cent. more, muft
neceffarily have reduced the brewery to a
fituation to which few other profeffions
are liable; becaufe moft manufactories
advance the price of the commodity in
proportion to the advance on the materials, a circumftance which can rarely take
place in the brewing bufinefs. The barley from Bremen, mentioned in the fecond
article, though apparently much inferior
to the preceding, was nearly equal in produce; becaufe it germinated freely, whilft
a great part of the other remained unmalted. And this accounts for the Norfolk

folk barley of that year having a real superiority. It was gathered in so much better order than the barley of the northern counties, which was in a great measure spoiled, that opposing the best of both sorts to each other, it was both superior in appearance and produce. From a similar cause, there appears less difference between the two seasons of the blown malt of Hertfordshire than in the rest, for the southern situation of that county is generally more favourable to the husbandman, in gathering the fruits of his labour, than can be expected in the more northern counties.

The last season (1783) though yielding a providential relief, was still very inadequate to the supply of the distressing deficiency caused by the preceding year. The backwardness of the northern harvests subjecting them to the autumnal rains which took place after the southern counties had finished their harvests, did irreparable damage to the barley; whence the obvious difference between the produce

duce of that and the barley of 1781; though happily much fuperior to that of 1782. The falling off obfervable in the third article, arofe partly from the indifferent quality of the barley, which was fprouted and much injured by the weather; and partly from the want of attention or fkill in the maltiter; from which caufes it barely exceeded the fecond article, which was from very thin barley produced in the neighbourhood of Berwick upon Tweed, but which worked tolerably well upon the floor. It is alfo worth obfervation, that the deficiency in the brown malt of the fifth article, bears nearly the fame proportion to the quality of the pale, in the fourth, that it did on the fame occafion in 1781.

I wifh it to be here particularly noted, that the feveral fums of the fermentable matter extractible from different malts, as above ftated, are thofe obtainable in the *ordinary way of practice*; but that by a particular modification of the extracts, and regulation of the procefs of brewing,

an

an addition thereto may be made, well worthy the brewer's attention. It is impossible to say what may be the amount of this addition in every case, because it must necessarily vary with that variety of practice observable in various situations and circumstances; but this I may venture to assert, that the general adoption of that mode of practice, which is meant to be reserved for particular communication, would effect a saving in the consumption of malt, in this kingdom, of at least 5 per cent. without the smallest diminution of the respective strength of the liquor produced from it. And I am confident in the assurance, that the advantage here alluded to, is not the hypothetical conclusion of a visionary system, but the real, solid, attainable benefit, arising from a particular mode of practice, which I have successfully adopted for a length of time sufficient to warrant its reality; nor is it over-rated, in the general estimate, if I may be allowed to judge from a comparison of my own practice, with that of

Z   others

others known to me in different parts of the kingdom. I also make a reservation of the event of this comparison, for no other reason than the probability that its publication might not be deemed proper to meet the eye of every reader *.

From the foregoing premises may be drawn inferences very favorable to the general use of the saccharometer, in the brewing business; and should its reception be such as the importance of the subject seems to claim, I may hereafter be induced to recommend an apparatus for ascertaining the value of malt to the purchaser or maker, independent of the consumer; in order that the buyer and seller of that article may adopt a clear and explicit language, conveying definite ideas, which by common usage may become as familiar to each other, and as well understood, as the terms made use of by the importers

* I however think myself at liberty to declare, that from the barley of 1786, I have brewed pale malts, which have produced, by the practice here alluded to, 88 lb. per quarter on an average, and some have amounted to upwards of 91.

porters and dealers in spirits; the value of which, but for the use of a similar inſtrument, would be as vague and indefinite as that of malt now is, eſtimated by the barbarous teſt of maſtication, or the equally uncertain one of floating in water, productive of no clearer language than is couched in the very equivocal terms of *bad, flinty, ſteely, hard, ſtiff,* and their oppoſites, *good, tender, free,* &c. &c. to which no poſitive idea can be affixed, becauſe they are relative to no ſtandard of compariſon.

SECTION V.

Of eſtimating the VALUE OF MALT, *and of regulating the* LENGTH, *or eſtabliſhing a ſtandard ſtrength for beers of every denomination, by the fermentable matter extracted.*

FROM what has been ſaid in the foregoing ſection, it will readily be ſuggeſted, that as the value of malt ariſes entirely from the quantity of fermentable matter it produces, the language of brewers,

Z 2 adopting

adopting the use of the saccharometer, will be, that " this or that malt producing so " many pounds more or less per quarter, " is of course in that proportion more or " less valuable;" and if we establish 82 pounds produce as the standard of what is now termed *good malt*, and estimate it somewhat lower than the present- exorbitant price *, viz. at 41 shillings per quarter, for the sake of an easy calculation, we shall see that sixpence per pound is the value of the fermentable matter of malt, estimated at that price per quarter; and that, therefore, the proportionate value of the malts of 1781, quoted in the preceding section, will stand precisely thus:

per Quarter.

1. Good *pale malt*, from Lincolnshire
    barley - - - - - - £ 2 1 0
2. Indifferent ditto - - ditto - - 1 17 6
3. Good *pale malt*, from Norfolk barley 1 16 0
4. Ditto ditto from Bridlington barley 2 1 0
5. Good *brown malt*, from the same kind
    of barley - - - - - - 1 19 0
6. Ditto ditto from Ware *(blown)* - 1 8 0

* *The price in* 1784.

On

On this view of the real, intrinfic value of the above malts, which value is demon-ſtrable to as great certainty, and by as eafy a mode, as the ſtrength of ſpirits is afcertained, no farther comment is necef-fary than the ſimple obſervation, that the difference in the firſt and ſecond articles aroſe from the different ſkill of the diffe-rent maltſters by whom they were made; the inferiority of the third reſulted from that inferiority of the barley, the defects of which the beſt artiſt cannot ſupply; the fourth and fifth ſhew the diſadvan-tageous effect of drying malt brown, though of equal quality on the floor, and cured upon the ſame kiln; and the ſixth expreſſes the deficiency produced by the practice of *blowing* up three kernels till they nearly occupy the ſpace of four, the natural inference of which is written in ſuch broad characters as to preclude the neceſſity of farther diſplay; for " he who " runs may read."

To reduce into order this very great ·irregularity, and to eſtabliſh a ſtandard

by

by which the effential value of all malts might be eftimated, and that every relative of that eftimate might be reciprocally communicated amongft thofe interefted in the fale or confumption of malt, in clear, unequivocal terms, it would be neceffary to lay down certain rules, and to eftablifh a certain criterion of perfection, by which the quality of every fpecies might be immediately tried, and explicitly communicated, as foon as difcovered; in which bufinefs the term *par* being adopted by the dealers in malt, with the fame intention as that of *proof* has been by the dealers in fpirits; and that *par* being fixed at 70 or 80 pounds per quarter produce, the diftinction of fo many pounds above or below *par* would be as definite and comprehenfive to the former, as that of fo much above or below *proof* is to the latter; particularly if recourfe could be had to an apparatus fimilar to that intimated in the laft fection, to correct their judgment and corroborate their affertions.

As

As the mode of forming this estimate of the fermentable matter extractible from malt consists, at present, in knowing the number of barrels of wort extracted from it, and discovering how many pounds each barrel contains, we are thence led to calculate the aggregate or sum of the fermentable matter produced by the malt employed, and to divide that aggregate into so many portions, or equal parts, as we wish to have barrels of wort in a fermentable state, or barrels of beer after the fermentation is finished; thereby providing for the establishment of a certain standard, or uniform strength, let the quality of the malt employed be good or bad. Hence, if the brewer has generally been accustomed to the use of indifferent malt, and should become possessed of some of superior quality, he may, at a certainty, reap every advantage accruing from that superiority, and not blindly waste it in a superfluous strength of his liquor; or, if he has commonly used good malt, and should accidentally purchase or

make

make a parcel of inferior quality, he needs not rifque the lofs of his credit by an unforeseen or unintended diminution of that ftrength which the confumer of his liquor expects to find; neither of which can be avoided by the prefent random eftimate of *fo many barrels per quarter*, in lieu of the more accurate one, here inculcated, of *fo many pounds of fermentable matter per barrel.*

To accommodate this to the practice of every brewer, no general ftandard is neceffary; becaufe the criterion of perfection in malt-liquors, as in moft other articles of domeftic confumption, exifting principally in the tafte of the confumer, and that tafte being as various and indefinite as the complexions, inclinations, and manners of the deciding parties, it is incumbent on every brewer to fix upon that ftandard ftrength, or final fpecific gravity of his wort, which by experience he finds productive of the required ftrength of his liquor. For inftance, fhould he difcover, from a repetition of experiments,

founded

founded on his ufual mode of practice, that 25 pounds per barrel is the gravity which produces fufficient ftrength for his general trade, he is then to eftablifh that, in his own mind, as his ftandard ftrength, which he ought always to produce, and which he needs never to exceed; for, fhould the aggregate extract of his malt produce, on a divifion into the number of barrels ufually contained in his length, a fuperior gravity, only in the ratio of 1 pound per barrel, making 26 inftead of 25 pounds, he would lofe an attainable advantage of fixpence per barrel (at the price of malt above-quoted) if he did not make fuch an addition to his length, as fhould liquidate that fuperiority, and leave his wort in its ftandard ftate. On the contrary, fhould the aggregate extract, on a fimilar divifion, fall fhort of the intended ftandard, the length, in the prefent procefs, fhould be leffened by extraordinary evaporation, and, in the future, by lefs copious extracts.

A a From

From a transient view of this subject, a person might be led to imagine, that if 80 pounds, for instance, are extracted from a quarter of malt, a length of two barrels per quarter would, of course, produce 40 pounds per barrel; that of two and a half, 32 pounds; and other lengths in the same proportion. This, however, would be a fallacious estimate. The quantity of hops used makes a considerable and perpetual variation herein; for though the dissoluble parts of that vegetable produce some addition to the gravity of the wort, yet the quantity imbibed by the hops exceeds the amount of that addition in so great a degree, as to make a considerable and irretrievable diminution in the aggregate of the fermentable matter extracted. But, in order to convey some idea of this matter, it may be observed, that the general product, by the general practice of the brewery, of what is termed *good malt*, is, upon an average, nearly as follows :

Burton

Per Barrel.

	Per Barrel.
Burton ale, of 36 to 40 gallons per quarter	40 lb.
Country ale, of 2 barrels — —	32 —
Ditto, of 2 barrels and a firkin ——	28 —
Ditto, of 2 barrels and a half —	26 —
Porter, of 2 barrels and a half ——	26 —
Ditto, of 2 barrels and three firkins —	24 —
Ditto, of 3 barrels —— ——	22 —

Thefe averages are, nevertheless, fo liable to variation, from the variety of proceffes adopted by brewers, and the various qualities of the malt made ufe of, that they are by no means intended as certain ftandards, capable of becoming a rule for general practice; though an occafional reference to them may not be unufeful.

But, to return to the regulation of the length, or final average gravity of the wort, I have to obferve, that as the amount of the diminution above-mentioned will be the fubject of our future difcuffion, I fhall here only intimate another difficulty which occurs in attempting to make the moft advantageous divi-

A a 2   fion

ſion of the aggregate extract into the intended proportions, and this exiſts in the incompetency of the ordinary prac- tice of the brewery to the obtaining *all* the fermentable matter which it is prac- ticable to extract from malt, the explana- tion of which is reſerved for the parti- cular communication before alluded to.

To remove, however, thoſe obſtacles which occur in the regulation of ſo much of the fermentable matter as is obtainable in the common mode of brewing, an at- tention to the following conſiderations is neceſſary, viz, that every wort to be aſſayed muſt previouſly be brought to that degree of heat which is eſtabliſhed as a ſtandard temperature for the inſtrument ; or a calculation muſt be made, to reduce it to that temperature, in order to deter- mine what its quantity and quality would be, when ſo reduced ; becauſe the expan- ſion, or increaſed volume of fluids of dif- ferent denſities, is not in the ſame ratio by the application of the ſame degree of heat, nor is the difference of their increaſe

creafe in proportion to their different denfities. To obviate this difficulty, I
have been induced to give, with the inftrument, the *Table of Expanfion*, which,
fhewing the degree of expanfion in worts
of different gravities, from 1 to 60 pounds
per barrel, enables us to afcertain the
different volumes of the fame quantity of
wort at different degrees of heat, from
50 to 200, by Fahrenheit's thermometer;
as well as the *Table of Heat*, before-mentioned, pointing out the difference between the apparent and the real value, or
fpecific gravity of worts of the fame variety, noted at every pound per barrel,
and at every degree from 50 to 100, by
the fame thermometer; which tables include every practicable denfity and heat.
To have extended this table beyond its
prefent limits, would have fubjected the
inveftigator to inconveniences which will
be mentioned hereafter.

Being enabled hereby to determine,
with precifion, the actual fpecific gravity of every extract, when at 50 degrees of heat, and to afcertain what
would

would be the precife quantity, at the fame temperature, fo as to calculate therefrom the number of pounds of fermentable matter contained therein; we are next led to confider how this aggregate of fermentable matter fhall be fo difpofed, after the action of boiling, and its fubfequent cooling fhall have taken place, as to produce the exact number of pounds per barrel, which I have eftablifhed as a ftandard, productive of the required ftrength in our liquor.

In extracting from the malt the requifite quantity of wort, the experienced brewer will not be at a lofs, but in the evaporation which takes place in the copper, efpecially where long boiling is required, the uncertainty is fo great that we can never be affured, by any rule hitherto known in the brewery, that we fhall produce the defired quantity, and are thence frequently led into great and difadvantageous irregularities.

To furmount this difficulty, were no hops employed, we need only have recourfe

courſe to the rule mentioned under the article *evaporation*, and eſtimating thereby
how much of the aqueous parts of the
wort ought to be evaporated, during its
continuance in the copper, immediately
calculate its required gravity at the moment of its being turned out. Thus, if a
wort containing 40 barrels, at a gravity of
30 pounds per barrel, were required to be
boiled down ſo as to produce 40 pounds
per barrel, in a fermentable ſtate, the portion to be evaporated muſt, of courſe, be
one-fourth of the whole quantity, or 10
barrels; but ſuppoſing 3 of thoſe 10 barrels to be the amount of the evaporation,
from the period of turning the wort out
of the copper to that of its being in a fermentable ſtate, the evaporation of the copper will be only 7 barrels. Whence dividing 1200 pounds, the aggregate of the
fermentable matter contained in the wort,.
by 33, the number of barrels to which it
is to be reduced in the copper, the quotient
will be ſomewhat more than 36; which
would indicate the ſpecific gravity the
wort

wort ought to have, when evaporated by
boiling to 33 barrels. As soon therefore
as the instrument (by a repetition of oc-
casional experiments) shews the wort to
be 36 pounds per barrel, it should be immediately *struck*, or turned out of the
copper, and the then quantity would
undoubtedly be 33 barrels, though, from
the great irregularity of a violent ebullition, the guaging rod could not have
ascertained the quantity at that time.

But since hops must be made use of,
we have to encounter fresh difficulties
arising therefrom. In addition to the
1200 pounds of fermentable matter, in the
case before us, there will be to include the
extractible parts of the hops employed;
from the sum of which is to be deducted
the quantity of wort imbibed by the hops,
or rather the amount of the fermentable
matter contained in the quantity so imbibed, and the difference will be the net
aggregate of the fermentable matter extracted; which divided by the standard
strength intended, the quotient will shew
the

the number of barrels producible therefrom. The application of the inftrument
herein will be precifely the fame as in the
cafe juft quoted, with the advantage of
proving the total incompetency of the
guaging rod ; becaufe the fpace occupied
by the hops, the amount of their abforption, and the ebullition of the worts, render all attempts to afcertain the quantity
by a guage nugatory and impracticable.

. Thefe confiderations feem to claim the
attention of every brewer who boils his
worts by time, particularly during fo long
a term as is requifite in the porter brewery;
in which the irregularity of length is fometimes very confiderable. If the end of decoction (exclufive of the purpofe of extracting the prefervative qualities of the
hops) be to evaporate a certain portion of
the aqueous parts of the wort, in order to
infpiffate and render more prefervable the
remainder, it appears quite indifferent
whether the obtaining that end, to the degree which the experience of the brewer
has fhewn to be neceffary, be effected in

B b one

one hour or in five hours. When once obtained, whether in a short or a long time, by means of a quick or a slow fire, by a violent or a gentle ebullition, the application of the saccharometer will assure the brewer that he needs neither err in his quantity or quality; " a con-
" summation devoutly to be wished" by all who are interested in the emoluments of large breweries.

To facilitate these several particulars, the average amount of the extract from the hops is hereafter ascertained in its proper place, and a *table of the quantity of wort imbibed by different quantities of hops*, is added to those before-mentioned, as given with the instrument; to which is likewise added a *table of measure*, reducing barrels of 36 gallons into those of 34, for the use of such persons in the country whose barrels are of the latter contents.

The utility of these tables will be obvious to those who are not expert at calculation; and to those who are, the saving
of

of their time and trouble will be fome recommendation of them.

From what has been premifed on the fubject of the theory and principles of the faccharometer, I prefume the reader will be fufficiently prepared to enter upon the practical part, to which I now proceed.

B b 2   STATICAL

STATICAL ESTIMATES

OF THE

MATERIALS FOR BREWING;

OR,

A TREATISE

ON THE

APPLICATION AND UTILITY

OF THE

SACCHAROMETER.

PART II.

Containing EXPERIMENTS *and* PRACTICE.

IN order to apply, in practice, the doctrines inculcated in the former part, it
may be neceffary to advert to the experiments upon which they are founded, and
to recur to thofe practical corroborations
which

which at once exemplify, illuſtrate, and eſtabliſh them.

For this purpoſe we will ſet the general proceſs of brewing before us, and note the application of the ſaccharometer in the ſeveral ſtages of its progreſs as they occur.

SECTION I.

Of applying the inſtrument to the ſimple Ex-
tract, or the WORT IN THE UNDER-
BACK.

SO ſoon as the *tap is ſpent*, or the wort all drained from the malt into the under-back, by dipping it with a guage we aſ-certain the number of barrels extracted; by taking the heat of it, we determine its ſtate of expanſion; and by preſerving a ſpecimen in the *aſſay jar*, we are enabled to diſcover its ſpecific gravity, the moment it is cooled to an experimentable degree

of

of heat *. In this bufinefs, as I have
before intimated, the circumftance of evaporation is of no account; becaufe the
wort is immediately pumped up into the
copper, and is fubject to no material evaporation, but what is the object of fubfequent attention. Its ftate of expanfion,
however, requires confideration; becaufe
the guage, taken as above, can only determine the volume, or number of barrels,
at the degree of heat which it then happens to contain, but does not fhew the
number of barrels to which the fame would
be contracted, at any of thofe degrees to
which the application of the inftrument
is neceffarily limited; and therefore, without this confideration, the quantity of
wort would be falfely eftimated, and the
aggregate acquired denfity, or fum of the

fermentable

---

* The reafon of limiting the degree of heat for
experiments to 100, is to prevent incorrectnefs in
applying the inftrument; for, at a higher degree,
the heat being lefs ftationary, an error might arife
from the decreafe which would take place during
the experiment.

fermentable matter extracted, would of
courfe be wrong.

This circumftance induced me to inveftigate the principle of expanfion, as relative
to the bufinefs in hand, by means of the
apparatus before defcribed, and to form
the table, on that fubject, before referred
to; by the affiftance of which we come
at once to the defired information. For
inftance, in a brewing of 24 quarters of
malt, my firft wort in the under-back was
32 barrels, the heat of which being 145
degrees, by Fahrenheit's thermometer, I
took out my fpecimen, and cooling it in
the affay jar, found its fpecific gravity to
be 28.25 pounds per barrel. On referring
to my experiments on the fubject of expanfion, I found that in a wort of that
ftrength, the amount of the expanfion at
145 degrees, is in a ratio of 1.69 per
cent. *i. e.* 100 barrels of wort of that fpecific gravity, and at that degree of heat,
would be 1.69 lefs in bulk, or only 98.31
barrels in the whole, when cooled to 50
degrees, fuppofing all evaporation to have
been

been prevented. Therefore, as 100 is to 98.31, fo is 32 to 31.47, which fhews that my 32 barrels, if fuffered to have cooled to the ftandard temperature of the inftrument, would have been only 31.47, or not quite 31 barrels and a half. To find the aggregate of the fermentable matter extracted in this wort, I multiplied 31.47, the quantity, by 28.25, the fpecific gravity, and the product was 889 pounds.

My fecond wort, from the fame malt, was 30 barrels, at 160 degrees of heat, and its fpecific gravity was 17.6 pounds per barrel. Making again the fame reference as in the former wort, I found that the amount of the expanfion of this wort was 2 per cent. and that, by the fame rule of proportion, my 30 barrels were only 29.4 at the ftandard temperature. Hence the product of that quantity of wort, multiplied as before by its fpecific gravity, was 517.4 pounds, the aggregate of the fermentable matter contained therein.

A

A third wort was 31 barrels at 170 degrees of heat, and its fpecific gravity was 9.25 pounds ber barrel; the expanfion of which amounting to 2.33 per cent. I found, by fimilar modes of enquiry, that there were only 30.26 barrels, the aggregate fermentable matter of which was 279.9 pounds.

Thefe aggregates being all added together, the fum of the fermentable matter extracted appeared to be 1686.3 pounds.

Without having taken into confideration the ftate of the expanfion of thefe worts, they would have ftood thus:

Wort.	Barrels.	per Barrel.		Pounds.
Firft	32	at 28.25	produces	904.0
Second	30	—— 17.6	——	528.0
Third	31	—— 9.25	—	286.7

Apparent fum of the feveral aggregates of the fermentable matter ——	1718.7
From which deducting the true fum	1686.3
The difference is ——	32.4 lb.

being the amount of the error which would have arifen from a calculation founded on thefe erroneous principles.

C ç   In

In conducting these experiments I had always the precaution to guage the wort, and take the specimen out of the under-back, as before recommended, just at the time the wort was about to be pumped into the copper, the mash-tun cocks being turned off. Had it been heedlessly guaged at an earlier period, the draining from the mash-tun, however inconsiderable in appearance, might have made too considerable an addition to the quantity to have passed unnoticed; and had the specimen been drawn from the last running of the wort, which is of a more dense consistence than the first, instead of being taken out of the under-back, an error of some importance, on the contrary side, might have been occasioned thereby.

The covering up the specimen in the assay jar had, also, been as carefully attended to, in order to be assured, that as it was at the moment of being taken out, an exact sample of the wort at that time in the under-back, though too hot to have

its

its gravity immediately afcertained, fo it might continue its faithful reprefentative when reduced to a lower temperature; for though an evaporation takes place during the time of its cooling, yet the vapour being confined by the cover, and prevented from efcaping, becomes condenfed by the coldnefs of the metal, and returning in drops, again mixes with the wort, which is thereby reftored to the fame ftate in which it was when firft put into the jar.

The refult of thefe obfervations being duly noted, I had only to wait the event of the fubfequent parts of the procefs, the inveftigation of which was as follows:

SECTION II.

Of the Effects produced in the Denfity of Worts by BOILING, *and by the Addition of* HOPS.

HAVING boiled the firft wort, abovementioned, its ufual time, I found that of the 31.47 barrels there remained only
21.5

21.5 when properly cooled; and on applying the inftrument to difcover its fpecific gravity, I perceived that it had increafed to 34.25 pounds per barrel. Multiplying, therefore, 21.5 by 34.25, the product of which was only 736.375 pounds, and deducting that fum from 889 pounds, the fum of the fermentable matter originally extracted, I difcovered a deficiency or apparent lofs of 152.625 pounds of that fermentable matter. Being well aware that this deficiency could not arife from evaporation, which, as before explained, can only carry off the aqueous particles, I was convinced that the abforption of the hops ufed was the true caufe of the lofs, which induced me to commence an immediate enquiry on that fubject.

In order to difcover what addition is made to the denfity of wort by hops, as a preliminary ftep to the difcovery of what they imbibe, I took half a pound of good Kent hops, and boiled them in water, as under:

Firft,

Firſt, in one hour, 12 pints of water were reduced to 7.5 pints, the ſpecific gravity of which was 1.75, or one pound and three-fourths per barrel.

2. The ſame hops in 12 other pints of water, which in one hour was evaporated to 9.4 pints, whoſe ſpecific gravity was 0.5, or half a pound per barrel.

3. The ſame in 12 pints more, which in the ſame time evaporated to 9.8 pints; the ſpecific gravity 0.22.

4. The ſame in 12 pints more, which in the ſame time evaporated the ſame amount as the laſt, and its ſpecific gravity was only 0.125.

From theſe experiments it is evident that the firſt extract is nearly two-thirds of the produce reſulting from four freſh applications of water, and as the hops uſed herein were in the proportion of 19 pounds to a barrel, in the firſt experiment, the extract of which was ſo inconſiderable as 1.75 pound in 7.5 pints, I thought the ſucceeding extracts too immaterial to be noticed in practice; for which reaſon, as

well

well as for conſiderations which will appear hereafter, I included the application of the firſt extract only.

The proportion of hops above-mentioned was thus aſcertained : As 7.5 pints, the quantity of the firſt extract, are to 0.5 pound, the quantity of hops uſed, ſo are 288 pints, the contents of a barrel, to 19.2 pounds, the proportion of hops per barrel, in this experiment. And the true ſpecific gravity of the firſt extract was thus found : I divided 19.2, the hops per barrel, by 36, the number of gallons per barrel, and the quotient 0.53 ſhewed the proportion of hops per gallon. Then ſaying as 0.5, the quantity of hops uſed in the experiment, is to 0.53, the proportion per gallon, ſo is 1.75, the ſpecific gravity of the quantity extracted, to 1.86, the true ſpecific gravity of the extract. Finding this ſo very near the proportion of 10 to 1, to avoid fractions, and unneceſſary references to tables, I eſtabliſhed it as a rule, that 10 pounds of hops will produce 1 pound additional denſity to the wort ; and accordingly for

300 pounds ufed in the wort above quoted, I added 30 to the fum of the fermentable matter (889) making in the whole 919 pounds.

I am not unapprized of an objection which might be made to the general eftablifhment of this calculation of the hopextract, on account of the irregularity which different lengths of time in boiling might occafion, and of the greater facility with which water may extract the diffoluble parts of hops, thence tending to invalidate this proportion as inapplicable to an extract made with a denfe wort: But as I have only taken the firft extract into my account; as other experiments of the fame nature have tended to eftablifh this proportion; and as its accuracy has been fufficiently confirmed by actual practice, it may be relied on to anfwer the purpofe of the niceft practitioner.

My next enquiry was directed to the difcovery of the quantity of wort generally imbibed by hops, in order to enable

me

me to account for the present deficiency, and to ascertain the amount of such as must necessarily happen in future.

I inclosed half a pound of good hops in a tin case, perforated with small holes, and sufficiently large for the purpose, suspending it by a string in the middle of a copper of first wort, which was suffered to boil one hour and a half. It was then hung up to drain till the inclosed hops were in the same state with those in the hop-back, from which the whole wort had drained. I next weighed a pint of the wort, when at a standard temperature, and found it to weigh 9862 grains net. The original weight of the hops (calculated at 440 grains per ounce, from the necessity of making use of weights so proportioned) was 3520 grains, which by the addition of the imbibed wort was increased to 25080. The dissoluble parts of these hops which must have been extracted, amount to 352 grains, according to the proportion above stated, which being deducted from 3520,

their

their firſt weight, there remained 3168
grains, being the then net weight of the
hops, independent of the worts actually
imbibed. I had now to deduct the ſaid
3168 grains, net weight, from 25080;
the groſs weight of the whole, and the
difference, 21912, was the true weight of
the wort imbibed by the hops; which
being divided by 9862, the net weight
of one pint, the quotient, 2.22 pints,
ſhewed the exact amount of the quantity imbibed by half a pound of hops.
According to this calculation, ſomewhat
leſs than 65 pounds of hops will imbibe
one barrel of wort, when well drained;
but, as the expedition required in practice will not admit of a ſcrupulous obſerv-
ance of every nicety, I find, from long
experience, that the average may be eſtimated at 60 pounds of hops, as generally
imbibing a barrel of wort; which eſtimate, alſo, from different experiments,
wherein meaſure inſtead of weight has
directed my calculations, is ſufficiently
corroborated and confirmed.

D d

Having

Having procured this information, I diſcovered that my 300 pounds of hops had imbibed 5 barrels of wort, which, at 34.25 per barrel, produced a deficiency of 171.25 pounds in the fermentable matter it contained; deducting, therefore, that ſum from 919 pounds, the aggregate of the extract of both malt and hops, I found that 747.75 pounds were all that could be expected to remain in the wort, at a fermentable temperature, *i. e.* when it had undergone the whole proceſs, fermentation only excepted.

On comparing this ſum with the actual quantity of fermentable matter found in the wort (736.375 pounds) there appeared ſtill a deficiency of rather more than 10 pounds; which may be accounted for by the probable ſuppoſition that there might have remained a ſmall quantity of wort in the hops, at the time they were returned into the copper, which would have drained out, had they remained a little longer in the hop-back. Eleven gallons

more

more would have effected the required
balance; and this, I prefume, is as near
an approach to fcrupulous accuracy as
is confiftent with the regular difpatch of
real bufinefs.

My fecond wort having boiled its al-
lotted time with the hops from the firft,
I perceived that the 29.4 barrels at 17.6
were evaporated to 22 barrels, and its
fpecific gravity was increafed to 25.5
pounds per barrel. Multiplying thefe together, the product (561 pounds) fhewed
that there was an addition made to the
fermentable matter of the fimple extract, amounting to 43.6 pounds. To
difcover how this could happen, I confidered that to the 517.4 pounds firft extracted, the hops carried with them, from
the firft wort, 171.25 pounds, which I
found they had imbibed, making in the
whole 688.65 pounds; but as they ftill
retained 5 barrels, the amount of the
quantity firft imbibed, I confidered that
the 5 barrels then imbibed, having difplaced the former 5, were only to be

eftimated

estimated at the rate of the specific gravity of the displacing wort; which being only 25.5 pounds per barrel, by multiplying that sum by 5, I discovered the amount of the fermentable matter then remaining in the hops to be 127.5 pounds, which, deducted from the gross aggregate, 688.65, shewed that the sum of the fermentable matter at that time in the wort should have been 561.15 pounds; and as the actual quantity appeared 561, the accuracy of this calculation is confirmed to a degree of nicety hardly to be expected on so practical an occasion.

Submitting to a similar process my third wort, the original quantity of 30.26 barrels at 9.25, was reduced to 20.5, at 16.5 pounds per barrel. These multiplied together shewed the sum of the fermentable matter to be 338.25 pounds, which exceeded that of the simple extract (279.9 pounds) to the amount of 58.35 pounds. Pursuing the same mode of investigation, I added the 127.5 pounds, brought into this wort by the hops from

the

the laft, to 279.9, the fermentable matter extracted, and the fum of them both was 407.4 pounds. Then deducting therefrom 82.5 pounds, the amount of the fermentable matter contained in the 5 barrels of this wort retained, at 16.5, (the fame quantity of the fecond having been difplaced thereby, as before) I found that the fum of the fermentable matter of the whole wort fhould have been 324.9 pounds, but in the actual produce (338.25) I found an excefs of more than 13 pounds, amply fupplying the deficiency of the firft wort; a cir-cumftance probably occafioned (as was before fuggefted) by a want of that time to drain from the hops, which the laft wort can always be allowed.

To render this bufinefs the more fa-miliar, I will recapitulate, and bring the whole into one point of view.

1. *Fermentable*

1. *Fermentable Matter extracted from 24 Quarters of Malt.*

			lbs.
First wort 31.47 barrels at 28.5lbs. per bar.			889.0
Second, — 29.4 —	— 17.6 —	—	517.4
Third, — 30.26 —	— 9.25 —	—	279.9

Total, 91.13 bar. at 18.52 lb. per bar. 1686.3

2. *Fermentable matter remaining after boiling the Worts, including the Extract of Hops.*

			lbs.
First wort 21.5 barrels at 34.25 lbs. per bar.			736.37
Second, 22.0 ——— 25.5		———	561.00
Third, 20.5 ——— 16.5		———	338.25

Total, 64.0 bar. at 25.55 lbs. per bar. 1635.62

3. *Calculation of the fermentable matter which ought to have remained, according to the preceding doctrine.*

First wort, produce — — 889.0 lbs.
Add, extract from 300 lb. of hops 30.0

———

919.0

Deduct, for 5 barrels at 34.25,
imbibed by the hops - - - 171.25

Carried over—*Net remainder* — 747.75 lbs.

```
                    Brought over  —  747.75 lbs.
Second wort, produce       —   517.4 lbs.
Add, fermentable matter brought
   in with the hops from the
   firſt wort      —         — 171.25
                                ────────
                               688.65
Deduct, for 5 barrels at 25.5,
   having diſplaced thoſe firſt
   imbibed      —             — 127.5
                                ────────
                 Net remainder  —   561.15
Third wort, produce     —   279.9 lbs.
Add, fermentable matter brought
   in with the hops from the ſe-
   cond wort   —              — 127.5
                                ────────
                               407.4
Deduct, for 5 barrels at 16.5,
   having diſplaced thoſe imbibed
   of the ſecond  —           —  82.5
                                ────────
                 Net remainder  —   324.9 lbs.

                 Total    —   1633.8 lbs.
```

4. *Correſpondence between the firſt and final ſtates of the aggregate fermentable matter extracted.*

Firſt State.

```
Sum of the extract from 24 quarters of
   malt contained in 91.13 barrels of
   raw wort  —   ‚    —        — 1686.3 lbs.
Extract from 300 pounds of hops  —   30.0
                                    ────────
                 Total   —   1716.3
                            ────────
                                  Final
```

Final State.

Sum of the fermentable matter contained in 64 barrels of wort in a
fermentable state —   —   1635.62 lbs;
Imbibed by, and remaining in the
hops, per calculation —   —   82.5

$$\text{Total} \;-\; 1718.12$$

By the foregoing state of the diffoluble
parts of the malt and hops employed in
brewing, we perceive, that however the
bulk of their containing vehicle be
changed, or their local or relative fituation
varied, the fum or quantum firft extracted
remains exactly the fame, fo far as we can
difcover by the means made ufe of for
afcertaining it. And that thofe means are
accurate may be readily inferred from the
confideration that the difference between
the actual and the calculated produce of
the 24 quarters of malt above quoted, does
not amount to 2 pounds in the fum of
1635; a degree of accuracy to which general practice can hardly expect to attain.

In

In the courſe of my own practice, I muſt acknowledge, the correſpondence, as above ſtated, has not always been ſo very accurate, the cauſe of which will be intimated in the ſucceeding ſection; but I am bold to affirm, that the reſult of my proceſſes, through a long and continued adoption of this ſyſtem, has ſo generally tallied with the principles therein inculcated, as to eſtabliſh and confirm the truth of them, beyond a ſhadow of doubt.

Having thus taken a general comparative view of the fermentable matter, in its origin and in the period of its entrance into a ſtate of partial annihilation, in the gyle tun, I come now to the particulars of its progreſs.

SECTION III.

Of the application of the inſtrument during the boiling of the wort, in order to RE-GULATE THE LENGTH, *or produce the ſpecific gravity intended.*

THE irregularity and inequality of the produce of the ſame quantity of wort

having

having been matter of frequent obſervation, I determined to enter into an inveſtigation of that buſineſs, with the view of eſtabliſhing the means of its prevention, on the ſure baſis of practice and experience.

At the time, therefore, that the firſt wort was going to be turned out of the copper, I took a quantity, filled an aſſay jar, and covering it cloſe, to prevent evaporation, ſuffered it to cool. I then tried its ſpecific gravity, and found it to be 31.76 pounds per barrel. Dividing this ſum in 736.37, the amount of the fermentable matter remaining in the wort, after the abſorption of the hops had taken place, the quotient 23.18, expreſſed the number of barrels of wort in the copper, at the period above-mentioned. The quantity of the cold wort, 21.5 barrels, being deducted from this, the remainder, 1.68, ſhewed the amount of the evaporation, or the quantity of wort evaporated, in paſſing from the copper to the cooler, including its continuance therein.

Proceeding

Proceeding in the fame manner with the fecond wort, I found its fpecific gravity, at the period above indicated, to be 23.46 pounds per barrel; which being divided in 561, the final aggregate fermentable matter contained in the wort, the quotient was 23.91 barrels, being the quantity of wort then in the copper. Deducting from this the quantity of the cold wort, 22 barrels, the amount of the evaporation appeared, by the difference, to be 1.91 barrel.

The third wort having undergone a fimilar procefs, its fpecific gravity proved to be 14.92 pounds per barrel; which being in like manner divided in 338.25, its aggregate fermentable matter, the quotient, or quantity of wort in the copper, at the above quoted period, was 22.66 barrels; from which having deducted 20.5 barrels, the quantum of the cold wort, the difference fhewed the amount of the evaporation to have been 2.16 barrels.

In order to make a general application of thefe difcoveries, I compared the three

evaporations

evaporations together, and found their relative proportions to differ confiderably,
as will appear from the fubfequent view
of them.

The firft wort of 21.5 barrels, at 34.25
pounds per barrel, had evaporated 1.68
barrel, which is in the ratio of 7.7 per
cent.

The fecond, of 22 barrels, at 25.5 per
barrel, had fuffered the greater evaporation of 1.91 barrel, or to the amount of
8.65 per cent.

The third of 20.5 barrels, at 16.5 per
barrel, had evaporated fo much as 2.16
barrels, or 10.5 per cent.

This comparative view fuggefted to me
the idea, that worts of different denfities
evaporate in different proportions, *ceteris
paribus*, and determined me to proceed in
fuch enquiries on the fubject as, being the
refult of prefent experience, fhould become the rule and ftandard of future practice, without having recourfe to the minutiæ of philofophical difquifition, which
the

the rude magnitude of my utenfils rendered inadmiffible or inefficient.

From a long and tedious courfe of experiments, which, I muft candidly acknowledge, did not always exactly correfpond with each other, I have been enabled
to form the *Table of evaporation* which
accompanies the inftrument, with thofe
before-mentioned, and which, I have no
doubt, will anfwer the intention of the
practitioner; having been formed with all
the accuracy and precifion of which the
nature of the bufinefs would admit, and
which a continued application of it, in my
own practice, has fufficiently confirmed.

That thefe experiments have not been
attended with all that correfpondent exac-
titude which philofophical precifion requires, is not to be wondered at, when we
confider the difpatch neceffary in actual
bufinefs, and the unavoidable irregularity
of thofe dimenfions on which our calculations muft neceffarily be founded.

In the firft place, if the guage of the
underback be not very correct, and its
contents

contents always dipped with the greateft nicety, the quantity of wort, and, of courfe, the fum of its fermentable matter, muft be wrong, and all calculations arifing therefrom muft be erroneous *ab origine*.

Secondly, if the quantity in the under-back be perfectly afcertained, and the affay jar, containing a fpecimen of the wort, be imperfectly or not at all covered, as there will be, in that cafe, an evaporation from the latter *, which does not take place, and therefore is not accounted for in the former, the real gravity of the wort, calculated from its condenfation only, will be wrong reprefented by it, and confequently caufe another error in the fum of the fermentable matter produced.

Thirdly,

---

* From fome curfory obfervations made on this fubject, it appears that the difference between a covered and an uncovered jar, is about 0.75 per cent. in a wort of 30 pounds per barrel and upwards; above 1 per cent. in a wort of half that denfity; and 3 per cent. in one of 5 pounds per barrel.

. Thirdly, fuppofing thefe particulars to have been attended to, with all imaginable care, the correfpondence between the actual and the calculated aggregate of the fermentable matter may not be correct, from the unavoidable retention of a part of the wort in the pump, which conveys it from the underback to the copper; from fome fmall quantity which may remain in the latter, intermixed with the few hops which will generally be left at the bottom; from the want of time for the whole of the wort to be effectually drained from the hops; and from a quantity of wort which may, and frequently does, remain in the hop-back, retained by the irregularity of the bottom, the feeds and fuch parts of the hops as have paffed through the falfe bottom, or by the back itfelf not being fet with a proper current towards the part where it difcharges the wort into the cooler.

Fourthly, fhould none of thefe obftacles intervene (which can fcarcely happen) the feveral proportions of the whole volume,

which

which worts of different denfities evaporate, may not always correfpond, with
philofophical accuracy, to the notations in
the table; becaufe the expofure of a
larger furface will produce a more copious
evaporation in a wort of equal volume and
denfity, than that of a lefs; and even a
ftrong current of air paffing over it, will
have a fimilar effect, by ruffling the furface, and thereby carrying off a larger portion of the aqueous particles than would
have efcaped, had it remained in a ftate of
quietude. From a few obfervations made
upon the difference of effect produced by
the different evaporations of the fame wort
in an affay jar and in the cooler, it appears that the latter, in many cafes, increafes the gravity 2 pounds per barrel.

Laftly, the difficulty of afcertaining the
exact quantity of wort, and confequently
of making an accurate calculation of the
fermentable matter it contains, by taking
a guage in the coolers, is not the leaft of
the obftacles to be encountered in this bufinefs. In large utenfils, where a volume
of

of 20 barrels of wort does not, perhaps, lie more than an inch deep in the cooler, without particular care, there is a hazard, of making an erroneous eftimate of 1 to 2 barrels in that quantity, by dipping, or, taking the depth only; for if the rule or guage made ufe of be perfectly dry, and the wort cold, as it fhould be at the time of taking the guage, the furface will bend, as it were, inwards, following the immerfion of the rule, fo as to make a vifible concavity round it; and if taken out then, the part wet with the wort will fometimes be near one-tenth of an inch lefs than its real depth. On the contrary, if the rule be moift, the wort, attracted by the moifture, will afcend upon the rule as much above the level of its furface, as, in the former cafe, it was below it.

A due attention having been paid to thefe feveral particulars, in forming the *Table of Evaporation,* I have no doubt but its judicious application will enfure to the practitioner the defired fuccefs.

F f   To

To apply it, in practice, we must invert, in some degree, the experiments on which it is founded, and by laying down its proportions as certain data, then proceed to the calculation of the specific gravity finally required. For instance, had it been required to produce from the first wort, in the foregoing example, a length productive of the final specific gravity of 34 pounds per barrel, we must have proceeded to calculate the specific gravity it ought to have, at the point of being turned out of the copper, and by occasionally taking out a specimen, cooling, and trying it, during the boiling (in the manner hereafter particularized) we should have been able to have turned it out in that exact state which would have produced the desired effect. The calculation is thus made:

31.47 Barrels of wort in the under-back,
  at 28.5 pounds per barrel —   — 889 lbs.
Extract of 300 pounds of hops   —   30 —

                               919 —
Deduct for 5 barrels of wort imbibed by
  the hops, at 34 pounds per barrel   — 170 —

Net fermentable matter remaining   — 749 lbs.

                                   Then

Then divide 749 by 34, the gravity to be produced, and the quotient will be the final quantity of the wort at that specific gravity, *viz.* 22.0 bar. Add the amount of the evaporation, in the proportion of 7.6 per cent. * which on 22

barrels is   —   — 1.67 —

Total — 23.67 bar.

Which is the quantity of wort in the copper, at the time of its being turned out. This divided in 749 pounds, the net fum of fermentable matter, gives 31.64 pounds, indicating the fpecific gravity the wort ought to have had at the above-mentioned period, in order to have produced 34 pounds per barrel in the cooler.

This rule is general, and may be applied to all lengths, adopting only the proportion indicated in the *Table of Evaporation*, as correfponding with the fpecific gravity intended, inftead of the proportion here adduced.

F f 2   As

---

* This is the proportion which a wort of 34 pounds per barrel will have evaporated, according to the *Table of Evaporation*; therefore, as 100 is to 7.6, fo is 22 to 1.67, as above ftated.

As there may be fome, however, who may wifh to avoid all calculation, as much as poffible, and who might prefer a rough fyftem and random principle, if calculated to fave time, and come near enough the truth for general practice, I endeavoured, from a comparative view of my continued experiments hereon, to accommodate thofe of this defcription with fomething in their own way. For having obferved, in the example before us, that my firft wort gained 2.49 pounds per barrel in gravity, by its evaporation from the copper to the gyle-tun; that my fecond gained 2.04 pounds by the fame means; and that my third increafed only 1.58 pound, from a fimilar caufe; I immediately concluded that certain principles might be eftablifhed for the purpofes above alluded to, fufficiently fatisfactory for the mere man of bufinefs; and accordingly, after duly digefting the feveral refults of my own long practice, I fketched out the *Table of the increafe of the gravity of Wort, occafioned by evaporation in the cooler;* by the adoption

of

of which, the careful practitioner will not be subject to an error of more than a small part of a pound per barrel, in his intended gravity. In case of this adoption, nothing more is necessary than to deduct from the intended specific gravity, the corresponding increase of gravity in the table, and the remainder will be that specific gravity the wort ought to have when turned out of the copper. For instance, in the table against 34, is the sum 2.40, as indicating the increase of gravity, which being deducted from 34, the gravity intended, the remainder, 31.6, shews the specific gravity of the wort in the copper, which is only a difference of 0.16 less than that indicated by the more accurate calculation of the table before recommended*.

In

---

* Since writing this article, the table has been collated with, and corrected by the table of evaporation, so that it may be adopted with as great accuracy as actual practice can attain to, as will appear in the following section.

In order the more expeditiouſly to cool the ſpecimen of wort taken out of the copper, for the purpoſe of noting its ſpecific gravity, I cauſed to be made the *Refrigerator*, already deſcribed, the application and uſe of which being hereafter particularly treated of, I ſhall proceed to the conſideration of the wort in the coolers, preparatory to its being ſubmitted to the action of fermentation.

SECTION IV.

Of forming AVERAGE GRAVITIES, *in order to produce the certain foundation of* UNIFORM STRENGTH.

THE firſt wort, in the above-quoted example, being cool, I took the guage and ſpecimen, and found the quantity and gravity to be as before-mentioned. Had this been fermented alone, this ſimple proceſs would have been ſufficient to have indicated its quantity and quality; but as other worts were to be added to it, my experiment thereon was not final. I,

therefore,

therefore, proceeded in like manner with the fecond wort, and making a fuppofition that thefe two only were to be fermented together, I demanded the average gravity of the commixture. To folve this I added 736.37 pounds, the net ferment-able matter of the firft, to 561, the net fermentable matter of the fecond, the fum of which was 1297.37 pounds.—I then added 21.5 barrels, the quantity of the firft, to 22 barrels, the quantity of the fecond, and dividing their fum (43.5) in 1297.37, the fum of the fermentable mat-ter, the quotient, 29.82, fhewed the average fpecific gravity required.

In like manner I added together the feveral net aggregates of the fermentable matter of all the three worts, the fum of which, 1635.62 pounds, being divided by 64 barrels, the fum of their feveral quantities, I found that 25.55 pounds per barrel (the quotient) was the average fpecific gravity of the whole gyle.

To

To have confidered either of thefe averages as a ftandard, and to have endeavoured to produce it accordingly, I muft have recurred to fome of my former calculations on this fubject. In the firft cafe, fuppofing it to have been intended that the two firft worts fhould have been fermented together, and that 29.82 pounds per barrel was the average gravity required, I fhould have fuffered the firft wort to have been boiled its appointed time, without having examined its gravity till in a proper ftate in the cooler; having then found it to be 34.25 pounds per barrel, I fhould have proceeded to confider how far the fecond wort of 29.4 barrels, at 17.6 pounds per barrel (at that time in the copper) fhould be evaporated, fo as to have produced the average intended. For this purpofe, I fhould have made a fuppofititious eftimate that the two worts would be finally of equal quantities, and thence multiplying 29.82, the required average, by 2, and from the product 59.64, deducting the gravity of the

firft

firſt wort 34.25, I ſhould have diſcovered that 25.39, the remainder, was the
required gravity of the ſecond wort; but
the quantity of both worts not being equal,
this gravity is ſuppoſititious, ſerving only
to eſtimate therefrom the amount of the
fermentable matter imbibed by the hops,
in order to aſcertain the net remainder,
preparatory to the calculation of the true
ſpecific gravity required; whence, according to the manner juſt inculcated, I
ſhould have proceeded to have calculated
the gravity it ought to have on being turned out of the copper, finally to produce
that required gravity. For example,

In the under-back 29.4 barrels at 17.6=517.4 lbs.
Add, Sum brought in by 5 barrels of the
   firſt wort remaining in the hops, at
   34.25   —   — 171.25 —

                                  688.65 —
Deduct, Sum retained by the hops with
   5 barrels of this wort, calculated at
   25.39   —   — 126.95 —

Add, Net aggregate of the firſt wort — 561.70 lbs.
   Apparent net aggregate   — 736.37 —

               Total 1298.07 lbs.

             This

This fum being divided by the required average, 29.82, the quotient 43.53, is the number of barrels of which the two combined worts are to confift; deducting from this 21.5, the number of barrels in the firft wort, the remainder 22.03, is the final number of barrels in the fecond; which number divided in 561.7, its apparent net aggregate of fermentable matter, fhews the required final gravity of the fecond wort to be 25.49 pounds per barrel.

Then, to the final quantity of wort in the cooler   22.03 barrels.

Add, the amount of the evaporation, in the proportion of 8.7 per cent, (as per table) which on 22.03 barrels is   }   1.91

And the total quantity of wort, at the time of being turned out of the copper, is   }   23.94 barrels.

Dividing this in 561.7, the apparent net aggregate, fhews the fpecific gravity of the wort in the copper to be 2..6 pounds per barrel. Or, purfuing the fhort method before-mentioned, the calculation would have run thus:

Specific gravity required — 25.49 lbs.
Deduct, increafe of gravity by evaporation 2.06 —
___
Gravity of the wort in the copper — 23.43 lbs.
___

The difference in thefe two calculations, refpecting the gravity of the wort in the copper, being only 0.03 per barrel, it is a natural inference that for general practice, the latter, unfcientific as it appears, will be preferred, for the fake of eafe and expedition.

I come now to the real ftate of the brewing before us, *i. e.* the three worts being intended to produce one uniform liquor, by being blended and fermented together, my attention was directed to the certain means of producing the average gravity required for the whole gyle, on the principles here laid down.

Premifing that 25.55 pounds per barrel was the average gravity, I paid no regard to the gravity of the two firft worts in the copper, but fuffering them to boil

their

their proper time, I made the neceſſary experiments on them in the coolers, and, according to the calculation juſt adduced, found their average gravity to be 29.82, as before-mentioned. This I conſidered as the average of two-thirds of my whole length, and that the laſt wort was of courſe to ſupply the remaining one-third. I therefore multiplied 25.55, the required average gravity, by 3, the number of the worts, and the product was 76.65; from which deducting 59.64, the product of the average gravity of the two firſt worts, multiplied by their number, 2, and the remainder 17.01, ſhewed the ſuppoſititious gravity of the third wort, on a preſumption of its quantity being the one-third part of the whole.

I then purſued my former method of calculation to find out its true, final ſpecific gravity, and thence to deduce the gravity it ought to have in the copper, in order to produce the ſaid final ſpecific gravity in the coolers, *viz.*

In

In the under-back 30.26 barrels at 9.25=279.9 lbs.
Brought in by 5 barrels of the second
  wort remaining in the hops, at 25.5   127.5 —

                                          407.4 —
Retained by the hops, with 5 barrels of
  this wort, calculated at 17.01   ——   85.05 —

    Apparent net aggregate   322.35 —
Add, net aggregate of the two former worts 1297.37 —

                          Total   1619.72 —

Which total divided by 25.55, the required
average gravity, shews 63.4 to be the
number of barrels contained in the whole
three worts; from which deduct 43.5,
the contents of the first and second, and the
remainder 19.9, is the final number of
barrels in the third wort; which number being divided in its net fermentable
matter 322.35, gives 16.2 pounds, the
true specific gravity required.

Then, to the final quantity of the wort in the
cooler   —   —   —   19.9 barrels.
Add, the evaporation (as per table) of
  10.5 per cent. which on 19.9 is   2.08 —
And the total quantity of wort, at the
  time of being turned out of the   ———
  copper, is ——   — 21.98 barrels.

                          Which

Which fum being divided in 322.35, the net fermentable matter, indicates the fpecific gravity of the wort in the copper, as above, to be 14.66 per barrel; which, by the fhort fyftem before referred to, would have appeared thus:

Specific gravity required — 16.2lb.

Deduct, increafe of gravity by evaporation 1.57

Gravity of the wort in the copper — 14.63 lb.

This again exhibits an erroneous difference of 0.03 per barrel, from the former calculation; and this difference, as I have before fuggefted, will moft probably be difpenfed with, in the hurry of bufinefs, for the fake of the difpatch neceffary in the general procefs of brewing; nor, indeed, is a nearer approach to mathematical certainty to be generally expected, in a bufinefs conducted on fo large a fcale as that of the brewery, for reafons before explained. *

Had

* Vide Note, page 221.

Had two of thefe worts been boiled together, a practice fometimes adopted, nothing more would have been neceffary
than to have multiplied the quantity of
each by its gravity, and by adding the
products of both together, to have confidered their fum as the contents of one
wort, and to have proceeded as above indicated, for the production of the gravity
required.

If we compare the refult of thefe calculations with the actual ftate of the feveral
worts, we fhall find a little variation, which
is not to be avoided. According to the
real products of the firft and fecond worts,
their average gravity, as above fhewn, was
29.82 pounds per barrel, the fecond being
22 barrels at 25.5; but, by my mode of
calculation, the latter being 22.03 barrels
at 25.49, the former confequently appeared 29.79 pounds per barrel. In like
manner, the real aggregate quantity of
the three worts was 64 barrels, whofe
average gravity was 25.55 pounds per
barrel,

barrel, whilft the calculated quantity was only 63.4 barrels at 25.54 pounds per barrel.

The caufe of this fmall difference (exclufive of the irregular draining of the wort, before treated of) exifts in the impracticability of previoufly afcertaining the precife quantity of fermentable matter finally contained in the latter wort, which alone is to fill up the meafure of the calculation, and produce the required average. For inftance, I knew that my third wort contained 279.9 pounds of fermentable matter; I knew alfo that the 5 barrels of the fecond wort, brought into this by the hops, made an addition thereto of 127.5 pounds; and that the then grofs aggregate of fermentable matter was of courfe 407.4 pounds. Could this have remained entire, the calculation would have been fimple, and the average certain; but as I was convinced that the 5 barrels of wort thus brought in, would only be difplaced by as much of the prefent wort, fo that 5 barrels of this
would

would ftill be retained by the hops; and
as it was indifpenfible that its fpecific gravity, at the time of this retention fhould
be afcertained, in order to difcover what
portion of the fermentable matter would
be retained therewith, and, of courfe, what
would remain to be added to that of the
preceding worts, I had no other means
of obtaining this information, than by
eftablifhing a fuppofition that the wort in
queftion muft be, when in the cooler,
equal in quantity to one-half of two
worts, or to one-third of three; and that
its final fpecific gravity muft confequently
be deduced from a fuppofititious gravity
founded on thofe proportions. Thus, in
the example before us, I was under the
neceffity of fuppofing the quantity of my
laft wort to be finally equal to one-third
part of the whole, and as its grofs contents were 407.4 pounds, I thence calculated the fuppofititious gravity of 17.01
pounds per barrel, which reduced the fuppofed one-third to 0.6 barrel lefs than it
afterwards appeared to be; yet as this

H h　　　　　　uncertain

uncertain principle has only relation to the quantity imbibed and retained by the hops, it has so little effect upon the general average, respecting either quantity or quality, as scarcely to merit notice; especially as the general practice of the brewery aims at producing the worts as equal in quantity as possible.

These rules and observations having, I presume, sufficiently explained the means of ascertaining average gravities, I shall now proceed to point out the end and purpose of their establishment.

SECTION V.

The utility of establishing a STANDARD GRAVITY, *as conducive to the forming therefrom an estimate of the* VALUE OF BEERS *of different qualities.*

WERE it in the power of the brewer to dispose of his liquor at a price proportioned to the quantity of malt employed, or rather, according to the portion of fermentable matter it contains, estimated

ted from the price of the malt itfelf, the application of the inftrument, as above directed, would immediately lead to the value of beers of every ftrength, deduced by the fimpleft calculation, from their average fpecific gravities only; but fince almoft every fituation has its eftablifhed price and ftrength, which, being entirely local, have no reference or relation to the prices or qualities of the beers of other places, nor are fcarcely ever to be regulated by the coft of the materials themfelves, it will be neceffary to eftimate the local value of beers of different qualities, by the relative proportion which the ftandard gravity of the wort bears to the obtainable price of the liquor which experience has fhown to be producible from that ftandard.　Thus, if it were required to brew beer of a different quality, to accommodate different confumers, the required ftrength being once known, we have then to calculate, from the general ftandard gravity, the price at which it fhould be fold, in order to be propor-

H h 2　　　　　tionably

tionably beneficial with the sale of the
standard liquor; or, the price being limited, we have in that case to discover what
strength must be produced for that price,
to be beneficial in a like relative proportion. For instance, supposing 25 pounds
per barrel to be the general standard alluded to, and that the beer produced from
it sold for 25 shillings per barrel, clear of
the duty, which should not be included,
it is an obvious inference that the product of any other gravity would be proportionably advantageous, if sold at the
rate of one shilling per barrel for every
pound of fermentable matter it previously
contained. Hence, if forty pounds per
barrel were the required gravity, the
price ought to be forty shillings, exclusive
of the duty; or if the obtainable price
were limited to thirty-six shillings, or
any other specific sum, the proportionate
gravity or strength would be thirty-six
pounds per barrel, or such other gravity
as should be correspondent to the specific
price. In like manner, were the same
standard

ftandard to be eftimated at a different
rate, a fimilar proportion muft take place.
Thus, premifing the ftandard price to be
but twenty-three fhillings per barrel,
exclufive of the duty, we fhould fay, for
a required gravity of forty pounds per
barrel, as twenty-five pounds, the ftandard
gravity, is to twenty-three fhillings, the
ftandard price, fo is forty pounds, the required gravity, to 36.8 fhillings per barrel,
the required proportionate price. Or, in
the inftance of the price being given, fuppofing it to be thirty-fix fhillings per
barrel, we fhould then fay, as twenty-
three fhillings, the ftandard price, is to
twenty-five pounds, the ftandard gravity,
fo is thirty-fix fhillings, the given price,
to 39.13 pounds per barrel *, the required proportionate gravity.

The

---

* It may be fuperfluous to remark, that the fpecific gravity every where mentioned in this article,
is that of the wort in the cooler, at a fermentable
temperature.

The propriety and utility of theſe calculations will be obvious to every one who is occaſionally engaged in the production of ſtrong beers intended to bear different prices; and even in that of ſmall and table beer, they will not be undeſerving of attention.

According to our firſt ratio, we ſhould learn, that if we ſuffered our ſmall beer to be of a gravity exceeding ſix pounds per barrel, when ſold at the price enjoined by law, it would be a leſs advantageous branch than that of ſtrong; and were a table-beer to be demanded, we could immediately calculate the gravity it ought to have, as above inculcated, proportioned to the price we ſhould obtain for it; and that with a degree of preciſion to which the uſual vague mode of eſtimating ſo many barrels per quarter, can in no wiſe bear a compariſon, and which muſt totally put to ſhame that more vague and barbarous appeal to the palate, authoriſed by the board of exciſe, or aſſumed by its officers, in characteriſing or determining

the

the quality of worts, as a rule for their
conduct in the charge of the duties; or
rather, as a means of detecting frauds,
or preventing impositions upon the revenue.

SECTION VI.

Of the attenuation of the fermentable matter,
or an attempt to ascertain the STRENGTH
OF MALT-LIQUORS, *by a comparative*
view of their specific gravities, prior and
posterior to the action of fermentation.

IN order to ascertain how far the
apparent *strength,* or the *inebriating qua-*
lity of beers, fairly produced by fermentation, had a relation to the quantity of
fermentable matter attenuated by that
action, I proceeded to examine several
different kinds of malt-liquor, whose previous or average gravity had been duly
noted, and the result of that enquiry was
as follows:

Strong

Strong Ale.

N°.	Gravity of the wort in a fermentable state.	Gravity of the beer when transparent.	Gravity lost; or amount of the fermentable matter attenuated.
1	42.0	18.6	23.4
2	41.7	22.5	19.2
3	41.0	20.8	20.2
4	40.6	18.1	22.5
5	40.0	21.6	18.4
6	39.0	18.5	20.5
7	38.3	17.8	20.5
8	36.7	17.2	19.5
9	36.0	12.5	23.5

Common Ale.

1	32.3	13.9	18.4
2	28.0	5.1	22.9
3	27.7	6.9	20.8
4	27.0	8.5	18.5
5	25.2	11.5	13.7
6	24.4	9.7	14.7
7	23.5	7.6	15.9

Porter.

1	29.5	8.3	21.2
2	26.0	6.5	19.5
3	25.5	6.0	19.5
4	24.5	6.5	18.0
5	23.3	5.3	18.0

Table

Table Beer.

Nº.	Gravity of the wort in a fermentable state.	Gravity of the beer when transparent.	Gravity lost, or amount of the fermentable matter attenuated.
1	—19.4—	— 7.5—	—11.9—
2	— 9.4—	— 2.7—	— 6.7—

On taking a comparative view of thefe fpecimens, and obferving that the amount of the attenuation did by no means correfpond with the original gravity, or that different worts were not attenuated in proportion to their refpective gravities, I was led to conclude, that all my former conjectures on this fubject were erroneous; efpecially when I confidered that two liquors equally attenuated, tho' originally of very different gravities, had apparent ftrength, or inebriating effects more nearly proportioned to their gravities, than to the amount of the attenuation.

I i   To

To be affured of this, I put one beer gallon of the *ftrong ale*, No. 5, into a fmall ftill, and having drawn over one wine-quart (before the completion of which, the liquor which came over had, for fome time, been mere water) I found, by experiment, that the ftrength of the liquor thus diftilled, was 36.4 parts of 100 proof fpirit; or, that the compofition confifted of 36.4 equal parts of proof fpirit, and 63.6 of water. Then faying, if one gallon of ale produce 0.364 quart of proof fpirit, 36 gallons will produce 13.1 quarts; by which I difcovered, that an attenuation of fermentable matter to the amount of 18.4 pounds per barrel, produces 13.1 quarts, wine meafure, of proof fpirit.

I then took one gallon of the weakeft *porter*, (No. 5) the amount of whofe attenuation was 18 pounds per barrel, and diftilling, in like manner, one wine-quart, its ftrength appeared to be 37.3 parts of 100 proof fpirit, which was in the proportion of 13.4 quarts per barrel. So that,

that, in this experiment, the attenuation of 18 pounds per barrel, produced 13.4 quarts of proof fpirit; a quantity rather exceeding that of the former experiment, though the attenuation was fomewhat lefs; which I am inclined to attribute to fome little difference in the accuracy of conducting them; the former having boiled over at firft, which might occafion fome lofs of fpirit, though the liquor thus thrown over was carefully returned into the ftill.

Several other diftillations which I made, with various fuccefs, ferved to convince me, that though the quantity of fpirit produced, did not, in my experiments, exactly correfpond with the amount of the attenuation, in the ratio above-quoted; yet the relation between them was fufficiently near to warrant my opinion, that, by a diftillation conducted on a larger fcale, and with meafures more philofophically correct, it will be found that every pound of fermentable matter attenuated by the action of fermentation,

I i 2

will

will produce the fame quantity of proof fpirit, by diftillation, whether that attenuation has been effected in a ftrong wort of 40, or a weak one of 10 pounds per barrel.

My prefent experiments, which I muft acknowledge to have been too imperfect and inaccurate to juftify my founding a fyftem upon them, do indeed tend to a fufpicion that the attenuation of weaker worts, produces a fomewhat greater portion of fpirit than that of the ftronger. Thofe which I have noted are the following:

N°.	Gravity of the wort.	Attenuation.	Spirit produced
1	— 40.0 lbs. —	— 18.4 lbs.	— 13.1 quarts
2	— 23.3 — —	— 18.0 —	— 13.4 —
3	— 25.2 — —	— 13.7 —	— 11.6 —
4	— 19.4 — —	— 11.9 —	— 9.7 —
5	— 9.4 — —	— 6.7 —	— 6.5 —

Now if we eftablifh the fecond experiment as a ftandard (having been the beft conducted) and calculate the proportionate quantity of fpirit producible from the feveral attenuations of the other experiments, they will ftand thus:

No

N°.	*Gravity.*	*Attenuation.*	*Spirit produced.*	*Spirit producible in the ratio of the second experiment.*
1	40.0 lbs.	18.4 lbs.	13.1 quarts	13.7 quarts
2	23.3 —	18.0 —	13.4 —	13.4 —
3	25.2 —	13.7 —	11.6 —	10.2 —
4	19.4 —	11.9 —	9.7 —	8.9 —
5	9.4 —	6.7 —	6.5 —	5.0 —

From this view of the fpirit actually produced, and the feveral proportions producible, according to calculations made from the quantity obtained by a very accurate experiment, it is evident that there is a correfpondent relation between the portion of fermentable matter attenuated, and the fpirit produced by fermentation, entirely independent of the original gravity of the wort, or the apparent ftrength of the beer, though that relation, as not immediately neceffary to my purpofe, I have not as yet had leifure to examine, with that accuracy and precifion requifite to eftablifh fo novel a difcovery.

In the inveftigation of this fubject there is, however, a circumftance prefents it-

felf

self to our consideration, of which I was not at first aware; and that is, the conviction, from these experiments, that *the apparent* STRENGTH *of malt-liquors, or that* INEBRIATING EFFECT *which they produce upon the animal frame, does not entirely consist of* SPIRIT.

To prove this, we need only advert to the experiments just noticed, where we shall see that ale so very strong as that produced from a gravity of 40 pounds per barrel, yielded no more proof spirit (the produce being strictly less), than the weak porter in the second experiment, of 23.3 per barrel; though the same person drinking an equal quantity of each, would have found their effects to have been powerful, rather in proportion to their respective gravities, than to the quantity of spirit producible from them. Indeed, if we consider the small portion of spirit contained in this strong ale; that it is not the one twelfth part of the whole; and that yet this ale (of the Burton kind) would produce as potent an effect upon the

the drinker, as the fame quantity of
fpirit and water, confifting of one fifth,
or at leaft one fixth part of the former;
we fhall be convinced that there is another principle in malt-liquors (if not in
all fermented liquors) befides that of *fpirit*, which contributes to that inebriating
quality to which common ufage has affixed the name of *ftrength*.

If we fuppofe this ftrength, in the prefent cafe, to be equal to a commixture
of fpirit and water containing one fixth
part of the former, we fhall then find that
this new principle is equal in effect to
the quantity of its concomitant fpirit;
for fuppofing each to be one twelfth part,
the fum of them both will be juft equal
to the quantity of real fpirit in the commixture above-mentioned, as their effects
are equal; and till we have a better clew
to direct our judgment herein, than the
fenfibility of the palate, or the ftrength of
the brain, we muft be content with probable conjecture, and rational hypothefis
for our guide.

The

The moſt natural ſuppoſition which occurs to me, on the preſent occaſion, is, that the principle here alluded to is the *gas* or *fixed air*, produced by, and inherent in all fermented liquors, ſo long as they contain the leaſt eſſential particle of their original compoſition, or of thoſe conſtituent parts which form their value ; and as the production of *inflammable ſpirit* is the criterion of vinous fermentation, and as that fermentation is always productive of the *fixed air* I am here treating of, it is a moſt probable conjecture that their production being concomitant, *ab initio*, ſo is their exiſtence inſeparable, ſo long as their laſt and leaſt characteriſtic particle remains.

That they are thus conſtantly and inſeparably attendant on each other, ſo long as the liquor which produced them merits our obſervation, may be eaſily demonſtrated. Simple diſtillation proves the exiſtence of the *ſpirit*, and the leaſt motion or cloſe confinement of the liquor ſhews that of the *fixed air*, by its inceſſant attempts

to

to efcape. Beer newly drawn from the cafk, or agitated in a glafs after remaining in a ftate of quietude, having by either means the coherence of one particle to another difturbed, is deprived of a confiderable portion of air, which is thence fet at liberty, and its efcape is vifible to the eye. The fame effect is obfervable after beer has been fome time confined in a bottle, by which means the perpetual tendency of the air to efcape is prevented; for no fooner is the cork drawn than the air rufhes with impetuofity from every part, to the furface, where its efcape is as fenfible to the fmell, as its progrefs thither is vifible to the eye *.

Its exiftence, as air, cannot be more incontrovertibly proved; and that it flies off with, or rather before the fpirit, in diftillation, there is not lefs doubt. The fmell difcovers its avolation and efcape before the fpirit is fufficiently rarefied to rife;

K k · for

---

* Air is fo abundant in malt-liquor, that if a glafs be fet in the receiver of an air-pump, on exhaufting the air out of the receiver, the air in the malt-liquor will rufh out fo violently as to convert the whole into a froth.

for being more volatile it muſt, of neceſſity, come over firſt; and the vapidity and
nauſeous flavour of the caput mortuum
which remains, after the ſpirit is drawn
off, ſeem to indicate that the fixed air has
taken its flight with its companion, tho'
the latter, only, is arreſted in a palpable
form.

Having thus demonſtrated that fixed
air is the conſtant attendant of the ſpirit
produced in malt-liquors, it remains for
us to endeavour to inveſtigate the cauſes
of its irregular produce, and to examine
its claim to thoſe effects which are ever
conſequent to that quality generally termed *ſtrength*.

Though in the inſtance juſt now ad-
·duced, I have ſuppoſed the fixed air and
the ſpirit to be equal, from obſerving their
united effects upon the drinker of the
liquor which contained them, and from a
compariſon of ſimilar effects produced by
a liquor of definite ſtrength, I do not
thence mean to inſinuate that they are always equal in quantity or effect, the contrary

trary of which is evidently the cafe; for the different proportions of either can only refult from accidents dependent on the previous ftrength or gravity of the wort, the mode of conducting the bufinefs of fermentation, and the manner of preferving the fermented liquor.

With refpect to the former particular (the gravity of the wort) we fhall be convinced of the inequality of the production of thefe two principles, by attending to the few experiments above noted. In the firft and fecond we fee the quantity of fpirit actually produced was nearly equal, yet the gravities of the worts were different in a ratio of 3 to 5, and the inebriating effects of the liquors, when fermented, were nearly different in a like proportion. Hence, taking it for granted that our firft experiment contained fixed air equal in effect to the fpirit which it produced, (*i. e.* one twelfth part of the whole) and eftablifhing that as a ftandard, we can calculate the real ftrength or inebriating quality of the fecond, according to the proportion

portion of its previous gravity, by faying, as 40, the gravity of the firft, is to 23.3, the gravity of the fecond, fo is 12, the fuppofed portion of fixed air in the firft, to 7, the proportionate quantity of fixed air in the fecond. Then adding the fpirit producible, according to the fermentable matter attenuated, to their refpective portions of fixed air, the ftrength of the two liquors will ftand thus :

Firft experiment, from the ftrong Ale, No. 5.

Spirit	- -	12
Fixed air	-	12
		——
Inebriating quality	-	24 parts of 144.*

Second experiment, from the Porter, No. 5.

Spirit	- -	12
Fixed air	-	7
		——
Inebriating quality	-	19 parts of 144.

Hence we fee that the inebriating quality of the fecond exceeded the proportion of its gravity, merely by an extra production of fpirit, the confequence of a different mode of conducting the fermentation ;

* *The number of quarts in a barrel.*

tion; for had the spirit produced been in the ratio of its gravity, the inebriating quality would have only been 14, instead of 19 parts of 144; for, as 40 is to 23.3, so is 24 to 14.

. If we try the third experiment by the same rule of proportion, we shall find that it falls short of the second, though from a wort of superior gravity, from the same cause which operated in favour of the latter, in the production of the extra portion of spirit just mentioned. For example, as 40, the gravity of the first experiment, is to 25.2, the gravity of the third, so is 12, the supposed portion of fixed air in the first, to 7.5, the proportionate fixed air in the third. Then estimating the producible portion of spirit (10.2 wine quarts) at 9 quarts beer-measure, the strength of the beer will be thus estimated:

Third experiment, from the common Ale, No. 5.

Spirit - - 9
, Fixed air - 7.5

Inebriating quality - 16.5 parts of 144.

Yet

Yet this, though it fell ſhort of the ſtrength gained in the ſecond experiment, exceeded the ratio of the firſt; for, according to that proportion, it would have been little more than 15.

We are hence led to the conſideration of the ſecond operating principle in this buſineſs, *i. e.* the mode of conducting the fermentation, which has a very conſiderable influence on the production of both the fixed air and the ſpirit.

In the firſt experiment, the great ſtrength or denſity of the wort requiring a greater force in the fermenting principle than was admiſſible in that particular practice which was to be productive of the qualities required in that particular liquor*, the portion of ſpirit was of courſe leſs than it might have been, if a ſtronger ferment could have been conſiſtently adopted. On the contrary, the ſecond experiment having had all the auxiliary force which can be applied to a fermentation intended to produce a potable vinous liquor, the attenuation

* Ale, of the Burton kind.

nuation of the fermentable matter exceeded
three-fourths of the whole, whilſt that of
the firſt did not proceed much further than
nine-twentieths, the conſequence of which
was, that extra-quantity of ſpirit obſervable
in the ſecond. And that the quantity of
fixed air in the latter was not equal to that of
the former may be attributed to the extraordinary force of the fermentation, which
carried off a great portion of it during its
action; for it is not to be doubted that
fermentation, conducted in a certain powerful manner, and carried to a certain length,
will ſo far deprive the liquor of its fixed
air as to render it ſcarcely diſcernible. It
may, therefore, be eſtabliſhed as a principle, that *the quantity of ſpirit produced
by an imperfect fermentation is leſs than its
fixed air; and that a fermentation carried to
its utmoſt length, diſſipates its fixed air in
proportion as it increaſes its quantity of ſpirit.*

A corroborating circumſtance, in ſupport of this principle, occurs in the deficiency of yeaſt, obſervable in conſequence
of an imperfect fermentation; for as wort
abounds

abounds in dormant, inactive air, inveloped in the fermentable matter, it is no sooner put into action than it seeks to disentangle itself, and in its escape becomes a doubly operative principle, *viz.* generative, in the production of spirit; and excretory, in the separation of the mucilaginous parts of the fermentable matter, which assumes the form of yeast; whence the more it is dissipated, the greater is its produce in these two articles, and *vice versa.*

The last particular which engages our attention, on this occasion, is the effects resulting from the manner of preserving the liquor. That this has an influence on the apparent strength will be generally acknowledged; but whether it is to be ascribed to an additional production of spirit, or to an increase of fixed air, or to a participation of both, I cannot take upon me to demonstrate, not having yet had opportunity to apply the still to the same liquor, at different periods, and in different modes of its preservation. I am, nevertheless, inclined to the opinion that the

generation

generation of the fixed air, as more obvious to the fenfes, is the more probable
caufe of that difference in ftrength diftinguifhable in malt-liquors kept in bottles,
though I do not mean to infinuate that
there is not a fimilar addition to the fpirit,
when kept in cafks, nor a partial addition
of each in both cafes. What I wifh to
demonftrate is, the certainty of the fact,
that fixed air is generated pofterior to the
completion of vinous fermentation; after
the liquor is become potable; and even
after accident or negligence has deftroyed
fome of its moft valuable qualities, and
rendered it unfit for ufe.

It is well known that during fermentation, the production of the fixed air is fo
abundant, that were not means provided
for its efcape, the ftrongeft veffels could
not contain it; and as the force of that
action abates, the avolation of the air proportionably decreafes, fo that when the
liquor is in a quiefcent ftate, the efcape
of the air is not perceptible. Yet after
the cafk is clofed, and it finds no other

vent

vent than through the pores of the wood, we frequently perceive it collected in such force as to rush out with great violence so soon as an aperture is made in the cask, and even to force a considerable quantity of liquor with it, to the height of five or six feet.

The same effect is observable on a change of the temperature of the external air, from cold to warmer, and that after the liquor has been for some months apparently quiet; for in this case, the fixed air being rarefied, escapes in greater quantity, and produces effects similar to those just described.

A further proof of the continual production of this air, is the *recovery* and *melioration* of beers which have been quite vapid and undrinkable, by the simple operation of bottling only. The cause of vapidity being nothing more than the total escape of the fixed air at that time generated, and the beer being thus deprived of its vital principle, can recover by no other means than those of an effectual

prevention

prevention of all further efcape, till fuch a portion of fixed air is again generated as will fupply the place of that which is loft. In that cafe, bottling is the moft efficacious remedy, particularly if the bottles are placed in a temperature fomewhat warmer than that wherein the cafk was, from which it was drawn. By this means the liquor, being ftill generative of fixed air, is again replenifhed with it, which effects its *recovery*; and that generative principle continuing ftill active, the air becomes abundant (all efcape being prevented) which is productive of *ripenefs,* commonly fo termed, or that *melioration* above alluded to.

It now remains for us to endeavour to fix fome criterion by which we may be affured that the fixed air thus generated, is a component part of the ftrength of fermented liquors. In this having unfortunately no better guide to direct our enquiries than the vague difcrimination of the fenfes, we muft be content to reafon from analogy, till fome further chemical

analyfis

analyfis fhall lay a foundation capable of fupporting a fyftem eftablifhed in mathematical certainty.

A judgment may be formed on this fubject, by comparing the different effects of equal quantities of the fame beer, one part taken from the cafk, when it is in a quiet ftate, and the other from a bottle, when ripe and full of fixed air; in which cafe, the apparent ftrength of the latter will be found fo far to exceed that of the former, as fcarcely to need any other argument in favour of the air we are treating of.

Of the powerful influence which this, as an inebriating principle, has upon the animal frame, I can fpeak from experience, and perhaps no inftance is more ftrongly in point than the following: Upon fome exhaufted, refufe raifins, from which wine had been juft made, I poured fome water, and after it had remained on them a fhort time, I let it drain off, when it was fo flightly tinctured, as to render it a matter of doubt whether the

water

water had imbibed a fufficient portion of the qualities of the raifins to produce the moft humble imitation of wine; for it was not difcoloured, but its tafte did juft imprefs a very faint fenfation of fweet upon the palate. It was, however, fuffered to remain till it became fomewhat tranfparent, when it was bottled, for the fake of experiment, without having exhibited any figns of fermentation; and after fome of it had remained two years, on being poured into glaffes, it exhibited every appearance of Champaigne, hiffed, fparkled, frothed, and threw up a brilliant fpray exactly imitating that admired liquor. Its effects were not lefs extraordinary; for they were inebriating in a degree nearly equal to thofe of Port wine, -though I am convinced there could not have been a portion of fpirit in the liquor equal to one-fiftieth part of the whole.

It may alfo be obferved, that bottled cyder, fretting wines, &c. produce fimilar effects from the fame caufe.

The

The gas, or fixed air resulting from the effervescence occasioned by the commixtion of acid and alkaline substances, is of this kind, as is evinced by the common mode of impregnating water therewith, in order to imitate that of Pyrmont, the apparatus for which is in the hands of most polite people. The effects of this air, without a particle of spirit, is a transient exhilaration (I will not call it *inebriation*) which passes off so much the sooner, on account of the total want of spirituous substance, and generative principle, in the fluid which produced it, to support its continuance.

To the same influence may be attributed the complaint of experienced topers, that they are sooner intoxicated by drinking different liquors, than they should have been had they drunk the same quantity of one sort, though equally strong. If mere spirit be the only efficient cause of intoxication, this commixtion of liquors could not produce the effect complained of; for, in that case, it would be indif-

ferent

ferent what liquor becomes the vehicle of
the fpirit, fo long as the quantum is the
fame. But this effect feems to originate
from the probable commotion and effer-
vefcence of the heterogeneous commixture
in the ftomach, producing or fetting at
liberty a quantity of fixed air, which
rifing into the head, is the affiftant caufe
of their complaint.

On the contrary, a fenfible diminution
of the inebriating effect is obfervable in
malt-liquors grown vapid or flat, agreeably to what has been before fuggefted
on that fubject. And that the caufe of this
diminution is the fame which occafions
their vapidity, *(i. e.* the lofs or efcape of
their fixed air) is evident from this confideration ; that the difference in effect is
producible in fo fhort a time as that of a
few hours, during which the expofure of
the liquor could not have produced any
perceptible diminution of the fpirit, tho'
it might completely have effected the
efcape of the fixed air, that being fo much
more

more volatile than the former as to be in a state of perpetual avolation.

If we recur to the sensations immediately consequent to the use of spirituous fluids, we shall perceive that those occasioned by a mixture of spirit and water are different from those which are the effect of strong malt-liquors; the probable cause of which is, that the strength of the former consists of mere spirit, and that of the latter is part spirit and part fixed air. The moment that a compound of spirit and water is taken into the stomach, it occasions a hot or ardent sensation; malt-liquor, on the contrary, excites first a gentle, genial warmth, which improves into a mild glow of the stomach and intestines, and differs from the former in the same degree as the warmth of the sun does from the heat of a fire.

It is not an improbable supposition that this difference arises from the different texture or consistence of the malt-liquor, whose spirituous particles are blunted or sheathed by the farinaceous mucilage with which

which it abounds; which alfo enveloping and being the efficient caufe of the fixed air, becomes the common medium thro' which both that and the fpirit muft act; whence that gentle fenfation of warmth juft mentioned, is the firft and only effect, till the heat of the ftomach has rarefied the air, and thence increafed its action and tendency to rife, by which means thofe confequent fenfations are effected. Hence thofe malt-liquors which are more abundant in fixed air, whether arifing from the materials or the procefs, are fofter upon the palate, and milder in their effect than thofe which have lefs, though the inebriating quality of both may be finally equal.

Thefe hints on the ftrength of malt-liquors, may fuffice for the prefent; and if they fhould be the means of exciting the curiofity and exercifing the talents of ingenuity to a farther and more effectual enquiry on the fubject, the purpofe of their publication will be fully anfwered.

M m   SECTION

SECTION VII.

PRACTICAL DIRECTIONS *for the general Application of the Instrument, in order to effect the Purposes before treated of.*

HAVING already pointed out the particular utility of the *Saccharometer*, in every particular stage of the brewing process, it may seem superfluous, perhaps impertinent, to a clear head and a comprehensive understanding, to enter into a detail of circumstances sufficiently indicated or inferred in the preceding sections; but since it may not be the lot of every one, who may wish to derive information and advantage from the contents of these pages, to be classed under that description; and as there are some particulars to be inculcated which have not hitherto been fully explained, I chuse rather to hazard the imputation of prolixity and repetition, than that of wanting perspicuity and precision, where beneficial information is intended

tended on a fubject never before committed to the prefs.

To anfwer the defired purpofe it is
neceffary to enter into the minutiæ of the
bufinefs, and to indicate the direct manner of effecting the intended information;
that every one, by clearly comprehending
the *means*, may with certainty obtain the
end.

The firft preliminary ftep to be taken is
the procuring correct tables of the contents of the under-back and coolers; the
former indicating the quantity contained in every inch of its depth; the latter pointing out the quantity at every
one-tenth part of an inch, and extending
to about four inches, deeper than which a
wort is feldom laid in the coolers.

A guaging rod is then to be provided,
fomewhat more in length than the whole
depth of the under-back, which rod muft
be graduated into inches, fubdivided into
tenths, or at leaft into fourths, which
latter divifion is in general fufficiently
minute for the purpofes of the under-

M m 2 back;

back; and where a small rule, divided into inches and tenths, is purposely provided for the coolers, there is no necessity for smaller graduations on the under-back-guage, if wanted for no other use, those being sufficiently near the truth for general practice.

The next thing necessary is a book, containing any number of leaves, of about the size of a half sheet of fool's-cap paper, ruled longitudinally into ten columns, for the purpose of a *diary* or *journal*; in which is to be inserted the particulars of every process, so far as they relate to the subject of which we are treating.

The first column is to contain *the date of the brewing*.

Second, the number of *quarters of malt used*.

Third, the *quantity of hops* employed.

Fourth, the barrels of *wort in the under-back*, the amount of the *expansion* being previously deducted.

Fifth, the *gravity of each wort* in the under-back.

Sixth,

Sixth, *the amount of the fermentable matter extracted* in each wort.

Seventh, the barrels of *cold wort in the coolers.*

Eighth, the *gravity of each wort in a fermentable state.*

Ninth, the *net aggregate of fermentable matter* remaining in each wort, at the above period.

Tenth, the amount of the *fermentable matter extracted from each quarter of malt.*

To thefe, as matter of not unufeful information, might be added two other columns:

The firft, to fhew the *fpecific gravity of the beer* in a ftate of quietude and tranf-parency.

The fecond, to indicate the *amount of the attenuation,* or the difference between the average gravity of the wort, and the gravity of the beer in the ftate juft mentioned.

In this journal our procefs before treated of, would ftand thus:

Date

Date.	Quarters of malt.	Lbs. of hops.	Wort in underback.	Gravity.	Fermentable matter extracted.	Wort in coolers.	Gravity.	Net ferm. matter remaining.	Ferm. matter per quarter.	Gravity of beer.	Attenuation.
1782.											
			31.47	28.5	889.0	21.5	34.25	736.37			
			29.4	17.6	517.4	22.0	25.5	561.0			
			30.26	9.25	279.9	20.5	16.5	338.25			
May 16	24	300	91.13	18.52	1686.3	64.0	25.55	1635.62	70.26	11.8	13.75

Sup-

Suppofing this brewing now to be proceeded upon, and that the faccharometer
and neceffary apparatus are at hand, fo
foon as the firft tap is fpent, and the mafh-
tun cocks are turned off, preparatory to the
fcond mafhing, we take out our fpecimen in an affay jar, and putting on the
cover, place it in the jar-cafe, before defcribed, premifing it to be already charged
with cold water; by which means it is
cooled, to an affayable heat, by the time
the bufinefs of mafhing is over. At the
fame time alfo, we note the heat of the
wort with the thermometer, and taking
the depth of it, with the guaging rod, we
refer to the under-back table of contents,
and againft the number of inches which is
the depth of the wort, we have the number of barrels it contains. But this, as
I have before explained, fhewing only
the quantity of the wort, in its then
ftate of expanfion, we make a minute or
memorandum of the quantity and heat in
any manner, to affift the memory, and fo
foon as the fpecific gravity of the wort is
found,

found, by the inſtrument, we have re-
courſe to the *table of expanſion,* according
to which we deduct the amount of the
expanſion, correſpondent to the heat and
denſity of the wort, from its apparent
contents, and enter into the journal only
what would have been the real quantity,
at 50 degrees of heat, ſuppoſing no evaporation to have taken place. Againſt
this ſum we immediately place its gravity,
regulated by the *table of heat,* and multiplying the one by the other, we find the
ſum or aggregate of the fermentable matter the wort contains; which ſum being
then inſerted in the next column, the
journal appears thus:

Date.	Quarters of malt.	lbs. of hops.	Wort in underback.	Gravity.	Fermentable matter extracted.	Wort in coolers.	Gravity	Net ferm. matter remaining.	Ferm. matter per quarter.	Gravity of tribe beer.	Attenuation.
1782:											
May 16	24	300	31.47	28.5	889.0						

N n

Pro-

Proceeding exactly in the same manner
with the second and third worts, we insert
them, in their turns, immediately under
the first, in the proper columns, as shewn
in the former example; and adding up
the several quantities of the three worts,
and the several sums of the fermentable
matter extracted, we divide the aggregate
sum of the wort in that of the fermentable
matter, and the quotient is the average
gravity of the raw wort; for instance,
91.13 divided in 1686.3 gives 18.52, the
said average gravity; which division is,
indeed, of no other use on the present
occasion, than by being placed in a line
with the quantity, gravity, and aggregate
fermentable matter of the whole wort, in
a fermentable state, to exhibit a comparative view of these particulars opposed to
parallel circumstances in the raw extract,
and thence to draw useful inferences not
inapplicable to future practice.

It generally happens that all the worts
in the under-back are assayed before the
first wort in the cooler is in a fermentable
state,

state, or sufficiently cool to be let into the gyle-tun; in which case the business of the raw extract, or wort, is entirely concluded, before that of the boiled is begun; and that, of course, the one occasions no interruption to the other.

Having finished and duly noted our experiments on this first part of the process, so soon as we find the first wort in the cooler in a proper state to let down, we dip it with our rule, graduated into inches and tenths, as accurately as possible, and take a specimen in an assay jar. We then refer to the table of contents calculated for the cooler, and noting the quantity correspondent to the depth which it happens to be, we insert it in the next, or seventh column of our journal, just as it appears, because the evaporation has taken place; after which, having found its specific gravity with the instrument, and rectified it by the *Table of Heat*, we note it in the succeeding column, and multiplying the one by the other, insert the product, or net aggregate of fermentable matter remain-

ing,

ing, in the next or ninth column, in the same manner as had been done by the wort in the under-back.

The second wort, when in a similar state, is submitted to the same process, and is noted under the first, in the proper columns of the journal, as appears in the former of the preceding examples. Should this, however, not be entirely cool, before it be necessary to attend to the third wort in the copper, it will nevertheless be generally so far advanced towards that state, as to be at an assayable degree of heat; and as the evaporation which takes place within the limits of those degrees, is not very considerable, we may venture to take the guage and specimen, and make our calculation, in the same manner as if it had been entirely cool.

If, however, in any instance, this wort should not be at an assayable heat, at the time we want to proceed to a calculation of the average gravity, the assay jar may be placed in the jar-case, to produce that effect. But it is to be remembered, that the

the jar is to be uncovered on this occafion, that fuch an evaporation may take place as the jar will admit, though, as I have elfewhere obferved, that evaporation would be very inadequate to the effect of the cooler.

This calculation of an average gravity I have before fhewn to be effected by adding the net aggregates of the two worts together, and dividing the fum by the number of barrels contained in them both, in order to difcover the average gravity of thofe two; which being confidered as the gravity of two-thirds of the intended gyle, we immediately proceed to calculate therefrom, in the manner before inculcated, to what gravity the third wort muft be evaporated, in order to produce the average gravity required in the whole. But this bufinefs having been already fully explained, in the third and fourth fections of this part, it only remains for us to indicate the mechanical or manual mode of producing the defired effect.

Herein

Herein we are primarily to confider how near the previous gravity of the raw wort approaches to the final gravity intended, and according to its approximation to or diſtance from it, to be earlier or later in our application of the inſtrument to the boiling wort, that we may not waſte our time by unneceſſary attention, nor our property, by a carelefs remiſſneſs.

A little experience will direct our judgment in this particular; for, by obſerving what portion of time is in general neceſſary to effect any given increaſe of gravity, we can, *ceteris paribus*, judge ſo nearly of the time requiſite for any other increaſe, as not to riſque an error, eſpecially if we are careful to begin our experiments a little earlier than we ſuppoſe it to be abſolutely neceſſary; a precaution not unworthy attention. Thus, if by experience we find that a gravity of 10 pounds per barrel, will be increaſed to 15, in three hours boiling, it would be adviſable to take a ſpecimen and make an experiment, after the wort has boiled two hours and a half;

half; and to adopt a fimilar precaution on any other occafion.

Thefe particulars being premifed, and the time recommended for making the firft experiment being arrived, we take the refrigerator; and having fixed on the perforated lid, we plunge it into the boiling wort. As foon as it is full, of which we can judge by its weight, we take it out, remove the perforated lid, put on the whole lid, and immediately immerfe it in a pail or tub of cold water of fufficient depth to reach nearly to the top, being careful that none of the water be mixed with the wort, by ruffling the furface, or caufing an undulating motion in it, on immerfing the refrigerator.

Having now the faccharometer, thermometer, and affay jar at hand, in about one minute's time, or a little more, the wort will be in an affayable ftate. This is beft known by flipping off the lid of the refrigerator, and applying the thermometer, at the end of that period; when (if we find the wort at an affayable degree

of

of heat) we immediately pour the wort
into the assay jar, and try the specific
gravity with the saccharometer; the whole
of which, as I have before intimated,
may, without the assistance of extraordinary dexterity, be effected in about two
minutes.

If by this experiment we find the wort
has not yet arrived at the gravity required
in the copper, we suffer it to continue
boiling, and repeat the experiment at such
intervals as our judgment indicates to be
necessary, till we perceive that our intended gravity is produced; at which time the
fire is to be immediately damped, or drawn
off, and the wort turned into the coolers.

When this wort is also cool, we take
the guage and the specimen, and finding
its quantity by the table, and its gravity
by the instrument, we insert them ordinal-
ly in the seventh and eighth columns of
the journal, under those of the preceding
worts; and multiplying, as before, the
quantity by the gravity, we discover the
net aggregate of fermentable matter it
contains,

contains, which we infert in like manner
in the ninth column. Then adding the
feveral quantities of the three worts together, and their feveral aggregates of fermentable matter, we draw a line, and
note their fums in their refpective columns; not neglecting to divide the latter
by the former, in order to difcover the
average gravity of the whole, which we
infert between the faid fums, in the column of gravity.

This being all that is neceffary to be
done refpecting the worts, we divide the
grofs fum of the fermentable matter produced, by the number of quarters of
malt employed, and the quotient fhews
the number of pounds of fermentable
matter extracted from every quarter of
malt, or the intrinfic value of it, which is
noted in the tenth column. In the example before us, the fermentable matter is
1686.3 pounds, which divided by 24 quarters, produces 70.26 pounds, the amount
extracted from every quarter ufed.

O o   At

At this period our journal, at a single view, and in one line, presents us with the following useful information:

1. The materials employed.

2. The gross value of the malt, indicated by the aggregate amount of the extract.

3. The net sum of the product of the materials; the specification of whose value comprises a plain definition of the quantity and quality of the whole wort, in a fermentable state.

4. The specific value of the malt explicitly defined.

If to these particulars we add the two columns above-mentioned, in that case we take the first opportunity of obtaining the gravity of the beer when transparent, and note it in the former; which being then deducted from the final average gravity of the wort, the difference (inserted in the last column) shews how much of the fermentable matter has been attenuated by the action of fermentation, intimating thereby the force of that operation,

ration, and its relative influence on the ftrength of the beer produced, according to the principles which have lately been the fubject of our inveftigation.

SECTION VIII.

INCIDENTAL CIRCUMSTANCES *in which the* SACCHAROMETER *may be of confiderable Utility.*

I have already had occafion to point out the ufe of the faccharometer in afcertaining the value of malts, but there are circumftances attendant on the ufe of it, in brewing, which, not being common, I have not yet mentioned. One of thefe is that difagreeable accident technically termed *fetting the goods*; which is the converting the malt in the mafh-tun into a pafty, clammy, gelatinous confiftence, by an injudicious application of improper heat in the liquor, or water ufed for mafhing, or from fome other caufe; the concomitant effect of which is a great deficiency in both the quantity and qua-

O o 2   lity

lity of the extract, in the detection of which the use of the instrument is singularly advantageous.

The occurrence of this accident *totally* is not, indeed, frequent; but I apprehend that its *partial* appearance is more common than many are apt to imagine. If the brewer knows how much liquor he turns upon the malt, he also knows what quantity of wort he should have in the under-back, if the malt be good, and the process has been properly conducted. Should this fall short in so large a proportion as one-third or one-fourth part, the goods may be said to be *totally* set; if in a less, they are *partially* set.

In either of these cases, if he estimates his loss by the quantity deficient, or attempts to make good the deficiency by a fresh application of water, on a supposition that his wort is strong, in proportion to the shortness of the length, or smallness of the quantity extracted, he is egregiously wrong. The instrument will shew him that not only his quantity
is

is lefs, but the ftrength or gravity of the extract is alfo deficient; from the difcovery of which he will be enabled to guard againft injuring the reputation of his beer, by a falfe eftimate of its ftrength, on that occafion, and will be prepared to provide for the prevention or remedy of fimilar accidents in future; for his lofs being accurately afcertained, the difcovery will naturally excite an enquiry as to the efficient caufe of it; and whether that be found to have exifted in the materials or the procefs, the experienced brewer will thence adopt a practice productive of better effects. This, however, is applicable rather to a *partial* than to a *total* fetting of the goods; for an accident of the latter kind will force itfelf upon the attention of the moft ignorant and carelefs, whilft there are degrees of the former which will efcape the notice of the intelligent and attentive, without the means of detection here recommended.

An

An accident of this kind once came within my own obfervation, wherein, by the inattention of a fervant, the goods were fo far *fet*, that by two mafhings, adopted to produce the ufual length of one, the gravity of the wort, which fhould have been thirty pounds per barrel, was only 11, and ftill the quantity was fomewhat lefs; being 31, inftead of 32 barrels; the lofs, therefore, in the firft extract only, may be thus eftimated :

	lbs.
Firft wort fhould have been 32 bar. at 30	— 960
Inftead of which, it was only 31, at 11	— 341
Deficiency	— 619

Which being divided by 75 pounds, the average amount of the fermentable matter then extractible from a quarter of malt, the actual lofs appears to be 8.25 quarters of malt.

In a fituation fo alarming, without the inftrument for my guide, I fhould have been totally at a lofs how to have proceeded, or to what purpofe to have converted a wort whofe quality muft have been

been unknown to me. Similar accidents, though in a lefs wafteful degree, I am convinced, do frequently occur and pafs unnoticed, in the want of thefe or fimilar means of difcovering them.

Amongft the caufes of fuch accidents may be reckoned the ufe of very low ground, and very high-dried malts, with improper degrees of heat in the liquor applied to them; and that of ftubborn, flinty, ill-made malts, and of fuch as are juft off the kiln, though attended with what would have been termed *proper heats*, on other occafions.

By the ufe of the faccharometer, alfo, we are enabled to detect that abfurdity in the practice of many country brewers, which the notable dames of yore agreed to call *leaking on*, a term which means nothing more than the continued fprinkling of water upon the malt, after the tap is nearly fpent, till the quantity of wort is produced which the brewer thinks will yield the required length, or quantity of beer, without any regard to

the

the quality of the malt, or that of the wort so produced.

The least reflection, without the aid of the instrument, will point out the absurdity, though reflection alone will not inform us how much is lost by the practice; for what power, or what time, has a fluid to extract, which is sprinkled over the surface of the materials, and immediately trickles out below, without being allowed a stationary moment for infusion? And though the practice I am here condemning is confined to some small breweries in the country, I cannot exempt the larger ones from all share of censure on the occasion; for if the *piece-liquor* of some of them is not exactly in that predicament, it verges so very nearly upon it, that I cannot pass it over without recommending the subject to the consideration of the proprietors.

Another circumstance wherein the utility of the instrument is obvious, is the being able to produce the same strength

in

in any malt-liquor, which we are defirous fhould be fubftituted for fome other, the produce of another place. If, for example, we would imitate Burton ale, Ringwood beer, or London porter, by being previoufly informed of the refpective average gravities of the worts which produce them, we can be correct in the imitation of their ftrength, a particular of which we cannot be affured by any other means; and this is of the greater importance, becaufe the malts made in one place frequently differ very much in quality from thofe made in another.

To exemplify this, I will fuppofe that a brewer of Edinburgh, being informed that the London brewery draws two barrels and a half, or two barrels and three firkins of porter from a quarter of malt, immediately fet to work, and drew a length in that proportion, without confidering the difference in the quality of the malt brought to the London market, and that produced in Scotland, we may readily fuppofe that he would find

P p   his

his liquor exceedingly deficient in point of ſtrength, and himſelf much diſappointed. On the contrary, if, being willing to make a random allowance for the ſuppoſed deficiency in the quality of the malt, he were to draw only two barrels per quarter, when perhaps it would have afforded two barrels and a firkin, he is then trading to a diſadvantage, which a knowledge of the ſtrength of London porter, and the application of the ſaccharometer, would have prevented.

By means of this inſtrument, too, the perfect analyſis of malt-liquor might, perhaps, be effected, with the view of diſcovering, with certainty and preciſion, the conſtituent parts of its ſtrength; and this diſcovery, by an ingenious hand, might lead to further advantages.

If the gravity of a given quantity of perfectly tranſparent wort * were taken, and

---

* It may not be unworthy obſervation, that wort in its natural ſtate of turbidity appears leſs denſe than when tranſparent; but the difference is very trivial. A wort of 49.75 pounds per barrel, in the former caſe, was exactly 50, when filtered through a flannel bag

and the portion of folid yeaft ufed to ferment it were exactly weighed; by taking
again the gravity, and noting the quantity of the beer, in a tranfparent ftate,
having previoufly weighed with precifion
the quantity of yeaft and lees produced
from it, perhaps a clue might be taken
hold of which might direct to the difcovery of the analytical procefs we are folicitous of. The amount of the yeaft and
lees, added to that of the unattenuated
fermentable matter, fhould make a fum
equivalent to the fum of the yeaft firft
ufed, and the amount of the fermentable
matter extracted; it would then remain
to be afcertained—how much fixed air
had efcaped during the fermentation—
what portion remained enveloped in the
unattenuated fermentable matter——the
amount of the fpirit generated—and what
portion of water made up the meafure of
the compofition *.

At

bag to perfect tranfparency; but not having had occafion to make any other experiments on this fubject,
I give it as the refult of one only.

* From curfory obfervation I find that a wort of
40 lb.

At least, the object seems worthy the attempt of any one who may have leisure, ingenuity, and inclination enough to undertake it; and should it not answer the end proposed, the enquiry is not incurious, nor unpromising of useful information; for, as Mr. Hales has well observed, " new experiments and dif-" coveries do usually owe their first rise " only to lucky guesses and probable " conjectures; and even disappointments " in these conjectures do often lead to " the thing sought for."

After what has been said upon the various, new, and useful purposes to which the faccharometer may be applied, I think it superfluous to dwell longer upon the subject; and therefore submit it to the reader to adopt or reject the use of it, as his own understanding may dictate.

APPENDIX

40lb. per barrel, though attenuated down to 12 or 13, does not produce of solid yeast and lees more than 10lb. per barrel, whence the quantity of fixed air escaped must, in such cases, amount to near one-half of the acquired density of the wort.

APPENDIX

STATICAL ESTIMATES, &c.

Defcribing the philofophical Principles upon which the Conftruction of the Saccharometer is founded.

By a FRIEND.

WHEN I tranfmitted you my firft notions of being able to procure a more accurate and compendious mode of making the *faccharometer* than what you had propofed, I only gave you the dawn of my ideas on the fubject. Having no foundation to argue upon but my own notions, I could not fpeak with that precifion neceffary for conviction. What I faid then, was only to fhew the propriety of your communicating to me all the information which you had collected from

your

your experiments, in order that I might know what there was a neceffity for my doing, and what I might let alone; but, perceiving that you were too much engaged to talk with me at large upon the fubject, and that, indeed, your experiments had not been adequate to my purpofe; being unable, alfo, to collect any kind of information in point from the paft inveftigation of the philofophical world here, I found there was an abfolute neceffity for my going through the whole of the enquiries upon the ground of my own examination; I was the more prompted to it, by obferving, in your reply to my notions and enquiries,

Firft, the impoffibility of vouching for the truth of a ftandard formed as yours had been. I do not mean fo much from the rudenefs of your guage and weights; for you will find, by a comparifon with what is contained in the following fheets, that in the weight of water you come near the truth; but from that flovenly manner of forming the firft ftandard wort, by

forty

forty diftinct *fillings* of a thing made of tin, which you call *a meafure*; where the error of every diftinct filling, of neceffity in itfelf important, muft, when multiplied by *forty* operations, grow into an enormous fize, unlefs that preternatural agency, called chance, was kind enough to extend its influence in the correction of one error by another.

Secondly, the appearance of a palpable error under which you labour, in the fuppofition of your prefent inftrument being perfectly the fame as it was before its accident;* and of which I think I can readily convince you. I will take it for granted that it was at firft, with No. 30 at top, the true reprefentative of the refiftance of a wort of 30 lb. per barrel, to the admiffion

---

* The accident here alluded to, was a bruife in the ball of the inftrument; which, in leffening the bulk of it by fo much as the bruife had indented or forced the metal inwards, made a lefs weight neceffary to fink the inftrument in water to the required point on the fcale.

admiffion of a body which, we will fay, contains 4 cubic inches;

Exprefs the weight of that cube by any No.　1000
Exprefs the weight of No. 30 at top by　—　100

Force exerted upon 4 cubic inches　　—　1100

Suppofe the inftrument, by a fimilar accident, or otherwife, to be leffened one-half, and become 2 cubic inches. In order to make it float at the fame point in water, you take off from the original weight one-half, and it becomes　　—　　—　500
Add the weight at top *unaltered*　—　　—　100

Force to be exerted, to fuftain 2 cubic inches　600

But the force with which your fluid is capable of acting on a cube of 2 inches, is only 550; and, therefore, will require an increafe of denfity in the relation of *
600 to 550, to fupport the inftrument with the addition of No. 30, again at 0;
and

* i. e. exactly double; this will be equally evinced by the more direct confideration, that the fame weight, added to a cube of 2 inches, and another of 4 inches, muft, in the former, require double the refiftance.

and in proportion as your preſent inſtrument has approached this diminution of its original cube, you are now making ſtronger wort than you did when the accident happened. It is true, that the weights are ſtill correct, that is to ſay, they are, in their relation to a fluid which will ſupport the inſtrument at o, the exact diviſionals of its reſiſtance; but the ſum of the reſiſtance is indubitably increaſed.

I have not a doubt that this mode of ſtating it will clearly indicate the exiſtence of an error; and that before you proceed with me through the following enquiries, you will be convinced, that the only method of rendering your inſtrument the ſame as it was, will be to reduce No. 30, and all its dependencies, till you reſtore the original relation between them and the cube immerſed.

It was upon theſe grounds, as well as upon ſome others of a leſs conſiderable nature, that I felt myſelf authoriſed in the ſuſpicion that there exiſted a partial fallacy in the very foundation of your ſyſtem.

But,

But, even suppofing it to have been accurately true, when I recollected the extreme difficulty and trouble which I found
in making with precifion the faccharine
mixture, at the time you were in London,
the fmalleft addition on either fide of the
required medium deftroying the intended
ftandard; added to the great indecifion
in noting any one accurate point upon
the fcale, owing probably to its attraction
to the furface of the fluid, I was clearly
convinced that an inftrument with its
ftandard weight being given for the
creation of future mixtures, by an immerfion in which to afcertain the weight
on the top of future inftruments, would be
extremely tedious in the operation, very
uncertain, unlefs conducted by a hand
which could be trufted to, and, if conducted by fuch a hand, expenfive. It is,
befides, to the laft degree clumfy and un-
philofophical, and fuch as one could hardly offer without a blufh to a workman,
who had a head capable of conducting the
businefs,

buſineſs, as the foundation of a new erec-
tion in the world of ſcience.

By all theſe reaſons, I was induced
to turn my thoughts to the procuring
a knowledge of the reſiſtance which
a wort, containing your propoſed ſtandard of 30 lb. per barrel, makes to
the admiſſion of a body immerſed in it,
compared with the reſiſtance made to the
ſame body by water; the difference of
which being aſcertained in figures, would
furniſh a preciſe, philoſophical, and eaſy
ſcale, upon which to form the relation between the inſtrument and its ſtandard
weight. This ſcale would have been ſupplied at once, provided the reſiſtance was
occaſioned by the force of gravity alone,
agreeably to the general axiom in hydro-
ſtatics, that *the weight of a fluid diſplaced
is always equal to the weight of the diſ-
placing body*; for, in this caſe, there would
have been no more to do than ſay—As the
weight of a barrel of water is to the weight
of any barrel of wort intended to be fixed
on as a ſtandard; ſo is the weight of the

Q q 2　　　　column

column of water difplaced (or its reprefentative, the difplacing body) to the famo
column of wort; the difference between
which would give the weight of No. 30.
But I was convinced, on reflection, that
there are other principles in fluids, by
which they refift the admiffion of a defcending body, and the firft of thefe is that
of attraction, which operating powerfully
on bodies compofed of heterogeneous particles, muft have confiderable influence in
fuch a fluid as wort. A tendency to co-
agulation in the higher temperatures, and
an approach to congelation in the lower
ones, which, perhaps, are only modifications of the firft, are certainly co-operating
principles in all gelatinous liquors; but,
as they probably have not much influence in worts, at leaft in thofe degrees
of temperature, within which you have
limited the examination of practice, I
confider only the operation of the two
firft, and to their combined effects I give
the

the name of * *ſpiſſitude.* It was my buſineſs then to enquire the relative amount
of that ſpiſſitude between the ſtandard
wort (of 30 lb. per barrel) and the ſol-
vent principle; which, being aſcertained
by the ſame weights, furniſhes the uner-
ring ſcale required.

In order to ſatisfy you clearly of the
truth with which this enquiry has been
conducted, and to warrant your confidence
in the adoption of this accurate foundation for your future ſyſtem, in preference
to the imperfect one, which was all that
your guage and weights had the power of
furniſhing you with, I ſhall enter into
rather a minute hiſtory of my mode of
conducting my courſe of experiments,
together with ſome account of the apparatus with which they have been made.

With ſome intereſt among the ingenious world here, I procured a ſcale beam
calculated to anſwer my purpoſes. I
found it would turn well with .03125, or

one

---

* I avoid the equally good appellation of denſity, becauſe common uſe has confounded it with
the idea of gravity alone.

one thirty-fecond of a grain (even with five
penny-weights on it) and fo ftrong as to
bear loading with four ounces troy, determinable then by 0.25, or one-fourth of a
grain.   To give it the command of the
latter, it was indebted to an invention of
my own, to take off the vibration ; which,
for accuracy and difpatch, I confider as a
very great improvement on the fcale beam.
My next thing was to *make* a fet of
weights accurately related to each other ;
finding upon examination that any which
could be purchafed ready made, were even
more erroneous than my opinion had firft
fuggefted.   By having accefs to a pair of
affay fcales, which would turn with $\frac{1}{100}$
of a grain, after a good deal of making
and re-making, I completed a fet of 11
weights in arithmetical progreffion from
1 to 1024 grains, and downwards to
.03125, or one thirty-fecond of a grain.
It was not for the fake of my experiments
alone, that I was at this trouble, my intention being at the fame time to furnifh
an

an accurate scale for the manufactory of future instruments.

To ascertain the relative gravities of different waters, being the first object, I got a very light phial blown of as large a size as my beam was capable, at the utmost, of supporting the weight of (nearly one-third of a pint). To the neck I joined a piece of a cylindrical glass tube, about $1\frac{1}{4}$ inch long, of a convenient size to admit readily of filling and emptying the phial. I afterwards ground off the top square, and also the inside of the neck, to some degree of truth; into this I fitted, by filing, &c. a fine cork, through which a small glass tube had been inserted and cemented, drawn at a little distance above the cork to the fineness of the smallest pin-hole, and there ground off. The cork I charged full of a composition of bees-wax and tallow, and finished it by a cement at bottom in a conical form upwards, to the aperture of the small glass tube in the middle. Around the top of the cork I cemented also a collar of wood, as a shoulder, to fit

square

fquare on the top of the neck which was ground off. This phial being filled near the top, and the ftopper, thus prepared, being introduced, the water, compreffed by the defcent of the ftopper in the cylinder, efcapes through the conical aperture; and the ftopper being preffed with care tight to the fhoulder, the water as it efcapes being taken off at the fmall aperture of the tube, gives an afcertained volume of water *, guaged to a very great nicety indeed. As a proof of it, in the commencement of my experiments, I filled it four fucceffive times with diftilled water, without varying at any one time one-fourth of a grain. I alfo refer you to the agreement of the three firft lines in the table of gravities, which were not fet down there until afcertained by the moft careful experiment.

* The quantity of water weighed being 2083 grains, and determinable then by 0.25, gives a guage to the $\frac{1}{8332}$ part of the whole, equal to $\frac{1}{10}$ of a pint, or about $\frac{1}{4}$ oz. per barrel; a degree of accuracy which you could not approach, and which I am of opinion would not be eafily exceeded.

ment. The procefs of each weighing was
as follows : I made a weight, which in the
oppofite fcale, ferved as an exact balance
to the bottle and ftopper, after it was
rinced out with diftilled water, and drained, but not too nearly, in order that I
might the more eafily, by adding or taking out a fmall portion of a drop, bring
it always on an exact equilibrium with
the weight. This operation of rincing
out with diftilled water and nicely adjufting, was patiently performed previous to every feparate weighing ; the phial
was then filled in the manner above defcribed, and from thefe operations is obtained the column of gravities as given in
the following table :

A Table of the *specific* Gravities and relative *Spissitudes of various Waters**.

	Gravity.	Spissitude.
Water, diftilled, *(by a common ftill)*	1000.	1000.
Ditto, ——— *(in pure glafs veffels)*	1000.	1000.
Snow, diffolved ———	1000.	1000.
Thames —— —	1000.3	1000.182
New River —	1000.3	1000.344
Chalybeate fpring, *Iflington* ———	1000.9	1000.889
Hare-Court Pump, *Temple* ———	1001.29	1001.349
Hard Spring, *Surrey* ———	1001.649	1001.664

In

* Since the firft publication of this treatife, the author has had opportunity of trying the fpecific gravity of various waters, in different places, of which the following are a part. They were fimply taken with his inftrument, and afterwards reduced to this fcale.

Peterfburgh, the river Neva —— —	1000.9
Dublin, well-water —	1002.178
Corke, river — —	1001.089
Drogheda, well-water —	1002.015
Belfaft, ditto —	1001.743
Dover, ditto ———	1001.498
Beverley, ditto —	1001.906
Newark, ditto ———	1002.069
Loughboro', ditto —	1001.443
Burton, ditto —	1001.361
——— another well ———	1002.178
Stamford, fpring —	1000.898
Wolverhampton, ditto —	1001.089

In order to examine the ſpiſſitude, I took the only one which was fit for my purpoſe of the various balls *, in the attempt to execute which, with propriety, I have been incurring a conſiderable degree of expence on your account, and from the diſappointment attending their being ſpoiled by various workmen hitherto, I have been experiencing a much greater degree of chagrin on my own. I fitted it up with a proper weight at the bottom, and a fine hair at the top, connecting it with one end of my beam, whoſe excellence furniſhed me by this means with a much more delicate hydroſtatic apparatus than any thing which could be procured, unleſs at a great expence. My mode of conducting the operation in each experiment, being that which is practiſed with every common apparatus of the kind, needs not be particularized to you ; it is enough to ſay that the difference between

R r 2   the

* Balls made for the firſt inſtruments.   J. R.

the weight of the fufpended ball in air, and its preponderation when immerfed in the fluid, gave me the meafure of the power exerted by that fluid in refifting the defcent of the apparatus, i. e. *the amount of its fpiffitude.* In this manner was the column of fpiffitude obtained *, to a perufal of which I now refer you, fo far as refpects the different waters †.

I

* The beam when the apparatus was immerfed in water having no more than 132 gr. about 5 dw. upon it, and turning with $\frac{1}{32}$ gr. afcertains the fpiffitude to a much greater degree of precifion than that with which the gravity has been done; for 1089, the weight of the cube in vibration, multiplied by 32, fhews the power of determining the refiftance of 1 in 34848.

† Neither the contents of the phial by which the gravity was afcertained, nor the cube of the ball immerfed to find the fpiffitude, could be fuppofed to be precifely 1000; but in order to furnifh a more immediate and agreeable comparifon between the relations of waters, &c. I have reduced all the fums, as given by my weights, to the fcale of 1000, by faying as the fpecification of the gravity and of the
fpiffitude

I had now got far enough in experiment to be able, from the *data* supplied, to know precisely, whether my notions of the necessity of this nice examination were warranted by the fact; and whether there really existed any other principles in fluids, besides that of gravity, co-operating in their resistance to a descending body. The reasoning on this is obvious; distilled water, if totally pure, I considered as a perfect homogeneous body, whose particles have no attraction to each other: I supposed ours perfectly so, and said,—as the gravity of distilled water is to its spissitude, so will the gravity of every fluid be to its spissitude, provided there be no other co-operating principle; but recurring to the table, and examining attentively the two columns, in a comparison between

spissitude of distilled water is to 1000, so are the specifications of all the rest to the sums inserted here. This method also gives, at one cross view, the immediate comparison between the respective gravities, and spissitudes, as will be alluded to presently.

between the water of the Thames and of
the New River, we find, in the former, a
deficiency, and in the latter an excefs of
refiftance. The fame is obfervable in a
comparifon drawn between the chalybeate
fpring and that of Hare-Court in the
Temple. I have alfo noticed the fame
phænomenon in a comparifon of other
fluids whofe gravities were nearly alike,
but whofe combinations were different;
from the refult of all which obfervations,
it might be amufing to the mind to lay
down theories with regard to the purity
or impurity of fluids, inferred from the
excefs or deficiency of that refiftance, compared with what they poffefs from the
power of gravity alone; but it is much
befide my prefent purpofe to purfue an
ufelefs train of fpeculation; it is enough
to direct you to a perufal of the table,
where the indication of a difference between the actual and comparative denfities of fluids, in proportion, perhaps, as
they confift of heterogeneous particles,

fhews

fhews the neceffity of attending to this circumftance, in the conftruction of an inftrument which is meant to meafure the relation between a fimple and a combined fluid *. It fhews evidently that a fcale formed on their comparative denfities, or, in other words, their fpecific gravities, muft be wrong; and that one formed upon their actual fpiffitude or refiftance, muft be clearly and indubitably right.

To the formation of this fcale I now proceed. And here I might have contented myfelf with getting your inftrument here, and examining the precife relation between it and its No. 30, by my weights, &c. have given that as a fcale upon which to form future inftruments; for whether your No. 30, as related to your inftrument, be or be not the reprefentative

* I fuppofe that the principle upon which the hydrometer for fpirits is conftructed, has been taken from the examination of gravity only; and poffibly the difference between real and comparative denfity, in fuch nearly homogeneous fluids, may not be fo great

fentative of an *accurate* refiftance of 30 lb.
of fermentable matter per barrel, is very
immaterial to the purpofe, fo long as the
amount of that refiftance is divided into
equal parts downwards, &c. But, as
I conceived it in fome degree neceffary,
in the formation of a new inftrument,
to give it a bafis which no philofophical
inveftigation can poffibly invalidate, and
being clearly convinced of the imperfection of your guage and weights for
the purpofe, &c. as I before noted, I
proceeded to enquire what the actual
refiftance or fpiffitude of a real wort, containing an addition of 30 lb. per barrel
was, compared with the actual refiftance
of water. The firft thing is to know
the

great as to render any other fcale neceffary for practice, although there certainly is fome difference in
the examination of philofophy. What that difference
is I would have enquired, but for reafons which will
be given hereafter; for I believe my apparatus delicate enough to have examined it with fome precifion.
To its fenfibility I am indebted for its having conducted me thus clearly to a proof of my firft fug-
geftions.

the weight of a barrel of water, which
is done as follows :

$$36 \text{ gallons in a barrel.}$$
$$282 \text{ cubic inches in a gallon.}$$

Cub. inches in ⎱ 231)10152 ditto in a bar. beer meaſure
1 gal. wine meaſ. ⎰

$$43.948 \text{ wine gallons in ditto}$$
$$58480 \text{ gr. Troy in 1 g. w. m}^*.$$

Val. of 1lb. ⎱
Averd. in ⎰ 7000)2570079.040 dº. in 1 bar. beer meaſ.
grs. Troy

$$367.154 \text{ lb. Av. in 1 bar. of water}$$
$$\text{Add } \quad 30. \quad \text{ſtandard incr. of gravity}$$

$$397.154 \text{ lb. Averd. in 1 bar. of}$$
ſtandard wort.

In

* The ſtandard addition to a barrel of water having
been fixed by you at 30 lb. Averdupois, I was oblig-
ed to go a little about, in multiplying by inches in a
barrel, beer-meaſure, and dividing by ditto in wine
meaſure, in order to reduce the former into wine-
gallons, that I might know its weight upon ſome
aſcertained ſcale, viz. grains Troy. The amount of
7310 per pint, or 58480 per gallon, being received
from one of the firſt enquirers into fluids here. The
water meant is rain-water.

The cubic inches in each are from examination
of *the ſtandards.* The number of grains Troy, per
pound Averdupois, is the relation of the two weights,
as lately ſettled by the Royal Society. It has long been
in

In the proportion therefore of 367.154 to 397.154 muſt my water be related to my wort, the comparative *ſpiſſitude* of which is to form the true relation between the inſtrument and its ſtandard weight.

To aſcertain this ſpiſſitude, which (from what has been ſaid above, in the diſcovery of the difference between the actual and comparative denſities of fluids) could only be done by examining the real fluid itſelf, I appealed to ſome minutes which I have of yours for the making of mild ale, and following the proceſs exactly, I manufactured a very well-flavoured wort, which I found about 5 lb. per barrel heavier

in eſtimation, varying a grain or two above and below that ſtandard.

☞ You make your water 369 lb. per barrel. The difference I impute to the imperfection of your guage and weights ; to the experiment being made in a half barrel, in which a ſmall error *plus* becomes doubled in the multiplication ; and to the circumſtance of your river-water being ſomewhat heavier than rain ; all which conſidered, I ſhould not have expected you to have come ſo near the truth.

vier than the propofed ftandard. I reduced
it afterwards with water, taking great
care to make the commixtion perfect;
and with much perfeverance and repeated fillings and weighings of my phial,
brought it exactly to the propofed ftandard 2253.336.

As 367.154, the weight of a barrel of water,
Is to 397.154, ditto —— of wort,
So is 2083.125 weight of my phial filled with di-
 ftilled water *,
To 2253.336, ditto — filled with ftandard wort.

The *fpiffitude* of which being immediately examined by the hydroftatic apparatus, and compared with that of the
original principle, I obtain the firft great
end of my purfuits, viz. an afcertained
fcale for the relation between the inftrument and its ftandard weight; for *as the*
S ſ 2
fpiffitude

* This calculation I begin from the ground of
diftilled or rain-water, becaufe it is fomething *precife
and afcertained*, and becaufe river-water, which is
in moft general ufe, comes fo nearly to it *(fee the
Table, oppofite Thames and New River)* as not to
make any difference in computation.

*spissitude of water is to the increase of spis-
situde, so is the weight of the saccharometer,
as floating in the same water, to the addition of No. 30, at the top, to bring it to
the same point in wort.* There needs not
any further illustration as a proof; but,
as a corresponding argument for practice,
I dismounted the ball of my apparatus,
adapted to it a weight at bottom, and a
regularly finished scale on the top, with
the notation of the point, o, as floating in
distilled water, making by this means a
regular saccharometer. Upon its immersion in my wort, and the addition of
a weight at the top, already prepared,
and now adjusted, agreeably to the accurate scale of proportion just obtained,
the instrument floated to the nicest precision at the same point, o, on the scale.

To complete the proportions of the instrument, there remained now only to
ascertain the size of that part of your addition to it, the sliding tubes, whose action was to counter-balance the difference
of density in all the different waters which
might

might come into officinal uſe in the
brewery, and with the conſtant variation
of which, in different ſoils and ſituations,
no ſingle inſtrument hitherto offered can,
otherwiſe than by accident, correſpond.
Recurring to the column of ſpiſſitude in the
table, I find the extent of this variation
in the variety of waters which I examined
to be 1.6 in 1000. The ſpring water which
exhibited the greateſt variation, (after a
confutation, by experiment, of imperfect
notions with regard to the denſity of
waters, which I had taken up from the
information of my ſenſes alone) was procured from a chalky, gravelly ſoil in the
county of Surry; and, from the experiment, as well as from the correſpondence
of the more domeſtic teſts of *hardneſs*, is
probably as much entitled to that characteriſtic as moſt in the kingdom. Sup-
poſing, therefore, 2 in 1000 to be the
limitation of the variation in ſpiſſitude between the pureſt water and any which
may come into uſe in the brewery, I went
to work with my hydroſtatic apparatus,
and,

and, by a little artificial increafe of den-fity, I made a water which correfponded with this proportion to the greateft degree of accuracy; by a comparifon of this with the fluid in its pureft ftate, I have afcertained the fize and length of the tubes, which are to compofe your regu-lator, in proportion to the ball: I have alfo, by this means, calculated the cube of the fcale, proportioned to the tubes, in fuch a manner as fhall, by notations upon it, indicate, on the firft immerfion in any water, the true adjuftment of the regu-lator, to the fmall divifional of 1 in 10,000 increafe of fpiffitude.

I was now furnifhed with every infor-mation neceffary for conftructing all the parts of the faccharometer; but whilft my hydroftatic apparatus was mounted, and before I threw away my wort, I thought I might as well proceed a little further, and by examining with a degree of nicety, which you will never be able to approach with the inftrument itfelf, the difference of fpiffitude or apparent ftrength at different temperatures, furnifh you

with

with a few correted points to recur to in
the formation of the tables, which muſt of
neceſſity accompany the inſtrument, in
order to aſcertain the true ſtrength of
worts under all the variations of apparent
value, from 50 to 100 degrees. An examination of the ſtandard wort at the two
extremes proved to me, in diret oppo-
ſition to what I had before imagined, that
the effets of heat are conſiderably more
ſenſible in the attenuation of fluids of a
greater than in thoſe of a leſs denſity, the
variation in this being 6.6, and that of
diſtilled water only 5.1 in 1000. This
unexpeted appearance ſuggeſted to me
the propriety of making a wort of 20 lb.
per barrel, and another of 10 lb. per barrel, in order to aſcertain as accurately the
extent of their variation. Having formed
them with as much preciſion as I had
done the firſt wort, I proceeded to examine
the whole three, at three equidiſtant degrees of temperature, viz. 50, 75, and
100; in order to note in each the gradations of ſpiſſitude, or apparent value.

From

From the refult of which examination
there occurs to me a difficulty in the formation of your tables of heat, which will
require much patience and perfeverance
to furmount. It arifes from the difcovery
of the following phænomena.

I. The expanfion of a fluid by heat between any two given points of temperature, 50 to 100, is conftantly
varying with the variation of denfity.

II. The expanfion between any two
mean points, 50 to 75, and 75 to
100, is alfo unequal.

III. At the time that the fum of the
expanfion between any two given
points, 50 to 100, increafes in proportion to the increafe of denfity;
in the intermediate divifions, between
the two points, it varies in a very
extraordinary manner; in the firft,
50 to 75, it increafes (though in a
different proportion from that of the
whole) with the increafe of denfity;
in the latter, 75 to 100, it decreafes
in an inverfe ratio.

I shall be better underftood by a reference to the following table; in which
from a nice examination of the fum of
fpiffitude or refiftance of various worts, at
different temperatures, the progrefs and
extent of this variation is exhibited at one
view.

*A comparative view of the extent of the
variation of fpiffitude, in liquors of different denfities.*

	From 50 to 75 degrees.	From 75 t 100 degrees.	Total From 50 to 100 degrees.
Wort of 10 lb. per bar.	1.703	4.132	5.835
Ditto - 20	2.315	3.782	6.097
Ditto - 30	2.87	3.731	6.601

From an attentive perufal of this you
will notice, that, owing to an irregular
combination of this afcending and defcending ratio, although the increafe of expanfion between any two given points in the
higher temperatures, is conftantly more
than between two equidiftant points in the
lower, (compare col. 1. and 2.) yet the
variation of this increafe, as the fluid increafes

creafes in denfity (viz. from 1.7 to 4.1 at
10 lb. per barrel, and 2.3 to 3.7 at 20 lb.
per barrel, &c.) is fuch, as to render it
utterly impoffible to give any calculation
from one wort which would be applicable
to another of a different value *, or to
fill

---

* A confideration of this will diffipate the remains of that regret with which, from other motives,
you were induced to give up your original fcheme
of fubftituting, in the place of thofe tables, the addition of another fliding tube to the inftrument itfelf,
whofe extenfion might counteract the variation of
apparent value, in the afcent through the higher temperatures. You will perceive that no fcale could
poffibly have been applied to it, which would have
correfponded with fuch irregular gradations of expanfion. It is from the clear evidence of this impoffibility that I was induced to take the trouble of examining an inftrument which has lately been offered
for the ufe of the brewery, under the recommendation
of a patent; in the appendage to which, from an ignorance of, or inattention to, the phænomena above
indicated, the inventor has been mifled into obvious
errors. I give you the detection of them at large, in
cafe you fhould think it of any moment to caution any
of your readers, whofe curiofity may have put them
in poffeffion of that inftrument, againft taking up
notions,

fill up the blanks between any two diftant points by any other means than that of tedious experiment. To purfue this enquiry thus, ftep by ftep, in all the degrees of temperature from 50 to 100, and through all the gradations, from the loweft to the higheft value of worts which a brewer can have occafion to examine, is a tafk of a very formidable nature; to undertake it, will require about half as much of refolution as its performance will of attention and patience.

It was my intention once to have attempted the purfuit of a fimilar enquiry with regard to fpirits, for the purpofe of

T t 2   forming

notions, with regard to your tables, from the evidence of fo fallacious a fcale.

** *The author is induced to fupprefs the publication of thefe detections. To point out the errors arifing either from negligence or miftake, is on all occafions an invidious tafk, and in the prefent is totally unneceffary. The mode of applying his inftrument is fo entirely his own, that it cannot poffibly receive a recommendation from the depreciation of any other. With regard to the accuracy of his Tables, he begs to refer to the teft of experiment.*

forming the relation between an inſtrument and its weights, upon a compariſon
of the difference of ſpiſſitude between alcohol and water; thereby furniſhing you
with the means of offering for the uſe of
the diſtillery the completeſt, if not the only
accurate thing of the kind that has hitherto
been conſtructed. By the exertion of a
little contrivance, the inſtrument, with
only the few weights it has at preſent,
ſhould ſerve in the double capacity of
aſcertaining the proceſs previous to the
operation of the ſtill, and of tracing the
preciſe value of the produce up to the
higheſt rectifications. In addition, however, to a variety of little obſtacles which
would occur here, in the execution of ſuch
an inſtrument, with a degree of accuracy
as ſatisfactory to me as that with which
the ſaccharometer is given, there is one
which it would reſt with you to ſurmount,
and which, I think, would ſtagger your
reſolution. The neceſſary toil of wading
through liquors, comprehending ſuch a
variety of denſity, in order to indicate the
real

real from the apparent value, at the different degrees of temperature to which
officinal practice might be accommodated.

Oppoſing to theſe impediments the limitation of ſale of ſuch an inſtrument, in
a circle ſo contracted as that of the diſtillery, compared with that in which your
preſent one is offered; and adding the
conſideration that it is not from the inſtrument itſelf that you propoſe to reap an
adequate compenſation for your labours,
I give up for the preſent our original
thoughts on this ſubject.

Should you, however, on any future
occaſion, reſume an intention of this nature, the ſame ſentiments which have
prompted me to fill theſe ſheets, induce
me to tell you that you may command
my beſt ſervices.

I ſhall be happy to hear that this hiſtory of my enquiries meets your appro-
bation, and am, &c.

London,
Jan. 24, 1784.

W. D.

The

The Uſe of the SACCHAROMETER *Simplified;*

*Or, The eaſieſt Method of applying that In-
ſtrument, in order to produce uniform
Strength in Malt-Liquors, without the
Minutiæ of long Calculations.*

ALTHOUGH I have the ſatisfaction
to find, that the calculations ne-
ceſſarily introduced in the practical part
of the *Statical Eſtimates* are ſufficiently
explicit and demonſtrative to the philoſophical and mathematical reader, yet having reaſon to believe that there are many
perſons in the brewing trade who may be
.deterred from the attempt to introduce
the ſaccharometer into their breweries,
on a ſuppoſition that it would be previouſly neceſſary to apply themſelves very
ſeduloufly, during a very tedious. length
of time, to the ſtudy of the ſyſtem inculcated in that treatiſe, even ſo far as to get
the whole of it by heart; and that,
after

after all, the calculations are of so complex a nature as to threaten inceſſant toil and unabating application, in order to accompliſh the deſired purpoſe; I have, therefore, thought it might not be unacceptable to this claſs of readers, to indicate the means of ſimplifying the general uſe of that inſtrument, by avoiding all calculations but ſuch as are indiſpenſably neceſſary, and would diſgrace a ſchool-boy to complain of.

This may be effected by dividing the principal buſineſs into the following heads:

I.

The mode of diſcovering the AVERAGE GRAVITY, *or* STRENGTH, *of ſeveral worts mixed together for an entire gyle.*

IN this buſineſs the brewer needs not to trouble himſelf with any thing foreign to his ordinary practice, except the taking a guage of each wort in the cooler, and the preſerving a ſpecimen in a jar, at the time he lets it run into the gyle-tun. As theſe

guages

guages are to be of ufe, he will, of courfe,
fee the propriety of noting them on a
piece of paper, or in any other manner,
in order to affift his memory at the time
that he may have leifure to apply them
to their intended purpofe. This may be
either on the evening of the brewing day,
or at any convenient time during the
next, but not later, particularly in mild
or warm weather; becaufe the fpecimens
taken out might begin to ferment fponta-
neoufly, if fuffered to remain longer, and
thence render the application of the faccharometer inaccurate. At this opportunity, then, the fpecific gravity of each
wort is to be taken with the inftrument,
and noted againft its refpective quantity,
as under :

Firft wort — 16 barrels at 35 lb. per barrel
Second　　— 18 ditto　— 21 lb. ditto
Third　　　— 17 ditto　— 12 lb. ditto

In all　51 barrels

Then, by fimply multiplying the quantity of each wort by its gravity, the fermentable matter they feverally contain is
indicated ;

indicated; and by adding their products together, the sum of the fermentable matter contained in the whole gyle is discovered. This sum being divided by the number of barrels of which the gyle consists, the quotient shews the number of pounds contained in each barrel, or the *average specific gravity* required.

In the present example we should say,
1st wort 16 barrels at 35 lb. make 560 lb.
2d ——— 18 ——— at 21 ——— 378
3d ——— 17 ——— at 12 ——— 204

In all 51 barrels, containing 1142 pounds

Which sum divided by the number of barrels, 51, gives 22.39 pounds; shewing that the average gravity, or strength of these three worts mixed together, is 22.39, or nearly 22.4 pounds per barrel.

This being discovered, the brewer must determine within himself, from the knowledge he has of his own trade, whether the liquor of which he has thus

U u ascertained

afcertained the fpecific gravity, be of fuch
a ftrength as to fuit the tafte of the confumer, and be thence confidered as a
ftandard, proper to be eftablifhed by him;
or whether it be neceffary to make any
addition to, or reduction of the fame. To
effect this, it will be neceffary for him to
proceed a ftep further, and confider,

II.

*How to produce, in a gyle confifting of feve-
ral worts, a given fpecific gravity, or
eftablifhed* STANDARD, *in order to effect
uniform ftrength in the beer.*

RECURRING to the average gravity
of his laft brewing, the brewer has only
to obferve how much that has fallen fhort
of, or exceeded his intended ftandard, and
to regulate his future practice accordingly.
For inftance, if it had been below the
ftandard, it would thence appear that he
had been too lavifh of his water; or if it
had been above it, he muft doubtlefs have
ufed too little.—The quantity, in either
cafe,

case, may be thus found :—Note the difference between the average gravity produced, and the standard intended, and
multiply that sum by the number of barrels in the gyle ; then dividing the product by the standard gravity, the quotient
indicates the quantity of water necessary
to be deducted from, or added to, that of
the next brewing of the same sort.

Suppose, for example, that the required standard is 25 pounds per barrel, and
that the last gyle brewed was 50 barrels at 23, instead of 25 pounds per barrel, which is, of course, two pounds per
barrel *under* the standard, or the beer is
so much weaker than the brewer intended. In order to remedy this inconvenience in the next brewing, premising
that the same kind of malt is used, we
should have only to say,

The present length — — — 50 barrels
Multiply by the deficient gravity   2 lb. per barrel
_____
Product 100 lb.

Which

Which is the amount of the fermentable matter wanting in the whole gyle. If, therefore, we divide this sum by 25, the required standard, we shall find, by the quotient, that there are four barrels of beer more than there should have been; which being deducted from 50, the number of barrels in the gyle, shews that there should have been only 46 barrels produced, instead of 50, and that if 4 barrels less of liquor be used in the next brewing, the beer, *ceteris paribus*, will be of the standard strength. The proof of this is very simple. If we multiply 50, the length, by 23, the strength of the brewing in question, we shall discover that there are 1150 lb. of fermentable matter contained in it. And if we multiply 46, the required length, by 25, the required standard, we shall see that this also would produce 1150, the number of pounds of fermentable matter which those 46 barrels would contain.

In

In the same manner, if the gravity of the preceding brewing had been 26.5, or 1.5 *above* the standard, we should say,

The present length — — — 50. barrels
Multiply by the superfluous gravity 1.5 lb. per barrel
_____

250
50
_____

Product 75.0 pounds
_____

Which is the sum of the superfluous fermentable matter in the whole gyle, or the redundant strength. This being divided by 25, the standard, the quotient 3, shews us that there might have been 3 barrels more in the length. In the next brewing, therefore, we should use so much more liquor as will produce 3 barrels of wort; and this addition, for brevity's sake, may be called 3 barrels, as in the foregoing example the surplus quantity is called 4; though every one can tell that a certain number of barrels deducted from, or added to, the liquor used for mashing, will not produce a reduction or addition

addition in the wort to the same amount, becaufe of the wafte in boiling, &c.

In thefe two inftances it is evident, that the former length fhould have been 46, and the latter 53, inftead of 50 barrels; a difference fo very material, that fcarcely any brewer will need to be told how much his intereft is concerned in attending to it.

The application of the inftrument, as here directed, fhould be invariably continued, in order that the brewer may be affured that he is working to his ftandard, as nearly as fuch a vague practice will admit; and in cafe of his ufing malt of a different quality, he needs only err in one brewing; in which, fhould the average gravity be either above or below the ftandard, he certainly can avoid a repetition of that error, fo long as he ufes the fame fort of malt, by applying the above fhort rules for its prevention. Should he, however, be inclined to endeavour at producing his ftandard gravity in the *firft* brewing of malt which he fufpects to be

of

of a different quality, I recommend to his confideration the following:

III.

Precautions to be taken on firft ufing a new parcel of malt, in order to produce the required ftandard gravity.

IT will be neceffary, on this occafion, that the brewer begin with the wort in the underback, in a brewing or two before he has finifhed his old malt, and make memorandums of the quantity and fpecific gravity of each wort; which memorandums are to ferve as a guide to his practice in ufing malt the quality of which he is not acquainted with. To exemplify this, I will fuppofe, that in the inftance quoted, the firft wort in the under-back was 20 barrels, at 30 lb. per barrel; the fecond, 22 barrels at 16; the third, 23 barrels at 9; and that thefe particulars were noted, for the purpofe juft mentioned, in the following order:

1ft wort 20 barrels at 30 lb. per barrel
2d ——— 22 ditto ——— 16 ditto
3d ——— 23 ditto ——— 9 ditto

In

In the firſt brewing from the new parcel of malt, let us ſuppoſe that the firſt wort proved to be 21 barrels; and that the ſecond wort was 22 only, as before; being now ſolicitous of knowing of what ſtrength they are, before we proceed to our laſt maſhing, we ſhould immerſe the jar with the ſpecimen of ſecond wort in cold water, as ſoon as taken from the under-back, in order to try it, the firſt wort having got ſufficiently cool by that time, without any immerſion. In two or three minutes the ſecond ſpecimen will be cool enough, when we apply the inſtrument to both, and find them to ſtand thus:

1ſt wort 21 barrels at 33 lb. per barrel
2d ——— 22 ditto — 18 ditto

The evident ſuperiority of ſtrength in theſe worts, over thoſe of the preceding brewing, from our old malt, muſt immediately intimate to us, that if we purſue our former practice, and maſh no more liquor at the third maſhing than we did before, our beer will be ſtronger than we require it. In order to liquidate that ex-
peoted

pected superfluous strength, we are to see
how much more fermentable matter we
have got in these two worts, than we had
in the two first worts of the preceding
brewing. We therefore say,

Former brewing, 1st wort 20 barrels at 30 lb.=600 lb.
     2d ——— 22 ——— 16 = 352
             In all 952 lb.

Present brewing, 1st wort 21 barrels at 33 lb.=693 lb.
     2d ——— 22 ——— 18 = 396
             In all 1089 lb.

From which deduct the amount of the former 952
            Difference 137 lb.

This difference is the sum of the superiority of the new parcel of malt over the
old, so far as we have proceeded; and as
our standard strength is 25 lb. per barrel,
we want to know how many barrels this
sum will amount to; which we find by
dividing 137 by 25, the quotient, 5.48,
shewing us, that we have an advantage
nearly equal to five barrels and a half of
beer, of our standard strength; and that
if we add five and a half barrels of liquor

      X x   to

to the quantity we should otherwise have
used for our third mashing, we shall produce the required strength, notwithstand-
ing we shall have so much more beer
than we had from our former malt.

This instance only relating to malt of
a superior quality, it will occur to the
intelligent brewer, that should his new
malt, on the contrary, be inferior to this
old, the same rule is to be adopted, in
order to find how much liquor he ought
to deduct from the quantity usually applied in his last mashing, as is here recommended for the discovery of the
quantity he ought to *add* to it.

IV.

*Directions for effecting the standard strength
in store vats, wherein beers of different
qualities have been started.*

THE practice above recommended is
also very advantageous in affording the
means of coming very near to the required standard, where several gyles of beer
are

are ftarted into the fame vat, becaufe he will have it in his power to correct the fuperfluity or deficiency of one brewing, by drawing a proportionate length in the next. It will be equally applicable to the producing the ftandard ftrength in a vat wherein the brewer may have put a quantity of beer of a fuperior or inferior quality; a practice which is fometimes found to be very convenient. In this cafe, it is only finding the difference between the ftandard and the gravity of the beer added, and multiplying that difference by the quantity; then divide the product by the ftandard gravity, and the quotient will difcover how many barrels muft be added to, or deducted from, the brewing which is to ferve as the means of bringing the whole to the ftandard required.

Suppofe 30 barrels of beer, of a former brewing, whofe fpecific gravity was 32, to have been ftarted into a vat, the gravity of which was intended to be 25 only, it is required to know what addition fhall

be

be made to the length of the next brewing, for that vat, in order to liquidate the superfluous strength of those 30 barrels?

Say, quantity of beer started   30 barrels
Superfluous gravity   7 lb.

Standard gravity 25 | 210 | 8.4 barrels

Hence it appears that 8.4, or nearly $8\frac{1}{4}$ barrels, must be added to the usual length of the brewing intended to be started into the same vat, for the purpose just mentioned.

As the same rule is to be observed in the instance of a quantity of beer being started of a quality *inferior* to the standard of the vat, in order to determine how much the length of the correcting gyle is to be lessened, it would be trifling to exemplify it.

———

THIS random mode of attempting the production of a standard gravity, how much soever I may be convinced of its utility to a certain class of men, I should

have

have been afhamed to have included in the foregoing treatife; and it is with concern that I intimate my fufpicions, that the majority of my profeffional readers will think the two or three rules here given abundantly fufficient for their purpofe, as well as a very competent fubftitute for the more elaborate fyftem I am folicitous of eftablifhing.

POSTSCRIPT,

POSTSCRIPT.

Containing PROPOSITIONS *for communica-*
ting the particular Application of the Sac-
charomer, alluded to in the firſt Part of
this Treatiſe, in order to effect a ſaving in
the Materials, from FIVE TO TEN PER
CENT.

TO fix poſitive terms for the particular communication of the means
of procuring thoſe benefits which are to be
derived from the Author's particular mode
of regulating the brewing proceſs, ſo far
as it concerns the application of the ſaccharometer, does not appear eligible, nor conducive to the end propoſed; which is, to
deter no one, by impreſſing the idea of
certain expence and uncertain gain, from
contributing, by his own experiments, to
render general a practice intended to be
productive of general utility.

As

As the probable advantages of this practice are confiderable, and as its difcovery was the refult of long application and laborious attention, the terms of communicating it ought to be liberal; but as its effects are various, according to the variety of procefs purfued by various brewers, a fixed fum, fuch as the author would chufe to accept, eftablifhed as a general premium, might be exceffive in fome inftances, and inadequate in others. The confideration, alfo, of certain payment, before the event of reimburfement or reward is afcertained, or rendered probable, would operate on the minds of moft people as preventive of their affent to a propofition apparently hazardous and problematical, accuftomed as men are to expect *value received* previous to their relinquifhing its equivalent. For thefe reafons, the Author propofes,

I. *To accept no premium*; but to reft his recompenfe upon the event of his practice.

II.

II. In lieu of fuch premium, a certain fpecific portion of the actual faving in the
confumption of malt, only, and that for
a limited time, to be fecured to him by
articles of agreement, which are to
include a claufe prohibiting the communication of the practice to any other
perfon, for a limited time, alfo.

In a compliance with thefe terms there
is no poffible rifque; and as no additional
utenfils would be neceffary, in a regular
brewhoufe, the practice may be relinquifh-
ed, without incurring expence or inconvenience, by any perfon who may be
blind enough to oppofe the darknefs of
profeffional prejudice, to the light of reafon and mathematical demonftration.

Further particulars may be learned by
addreffing the author, *(poft paid)* at his
refidence in HULL.

⁎ The SACCHAROMETER, in a ma-
hogany cafe, is fold by JOHN TROUGHTON,
Mathematical Inftrument-maker, Fleet-ftreet,
LONDON.

LONDON. Price *Three Guineas*, including the Book of Tables, and Directions for uſing the inſtrument.

Small POCKET THERMOMETERS to be had at the ſame place.

Thermometers of the ſize of thoſe above mentioned, are abſolutely neceſſary, where the brewer has none but the common large ones, uſed for taking the liquor in the copper, &c. which are generally too bulky to be introduced into an aſſay-jar; they are alſo equally uſeful for taking the heat of the wort in the coolers, as being more conveniently portable.

Country brewers may be ſupplied by means of their bookſellers, who have cor-reſpondents in London.

☞ It was the Author's wiſh, that the Gentlemen of the brewery ſhould have been accommodated with the Saccharo-meter at a leſs expence; but the difficulty of finding an artiſt capable of executing

Y y   a

a work of fuch extreme delicacy as that
of the *regulator*, wherein the pifton and
the tube, though both of metal, muſt be
perfectly *air-tight*; the length of time
requiſite to effect fo nice a piece of me-
chaniſm; and the tedioufnefs of regulating and adjuſting the weights and other
parts, to that correſpondent accuracy
with which he was folicitous the inſtrument fhould be finiſhed, and for which
every inſtrument executed under the di-
rection of Mr. Troughton is celebrated;
theſe conſiderations, maturely weighed,
will account for the neceſſity the inſtru-
ment-maker was under, of fixing the
price as above ſtated; and on a due reflection and compariſon of this, with the
price and execution of ſimilar inſtruments, now in the hands of the public,
it will doubtlefs be found but a bare
compenſation for fuperior workmanſhip
and fuperior correctnefs.

N. B. *Each*

N. B. *Each Book of Tables is numbered, correſpondent to the number of the inſtrument with which it is given, and ſigned by the author, as below; in order that the purchaſer may be aſſured of the authenticity of the former, and the accuracy of the latter,*

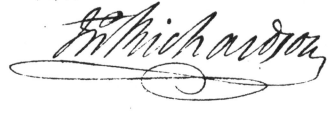

INDEX.

I N D E X.

A

B

Z 2   *Blown*

I N D E X.

Gas,

INDEX.

Gas,

INDEX.

G

H

J

L

M

INDEX.

I N D E X.

INDEX.

INDEX.

W

FINIS.

Made in the USA
Monee, IL
30 September 2022

14965403R00223